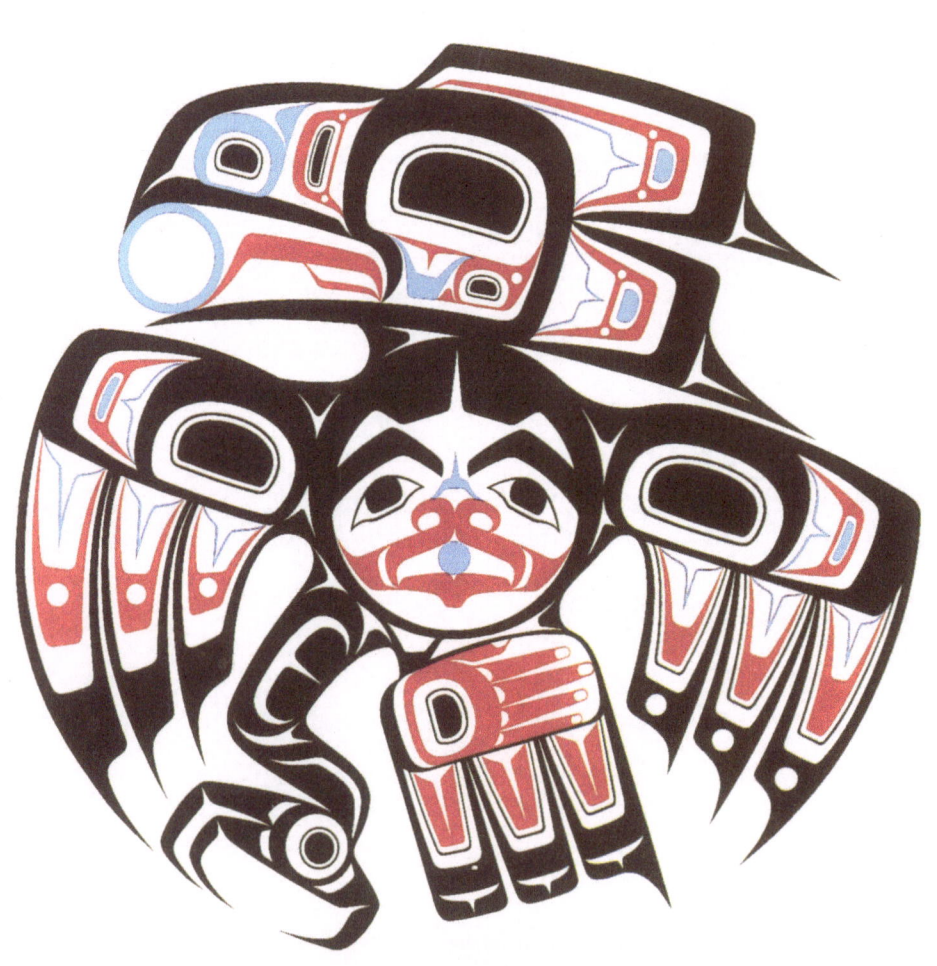

Non-Opioids in Pain Management

Vancouver, Canada, August 19, 1996

Edited by M.J. Parnham

Springer Basel AG

Editor:

PD Dr. Michael J. Parnham
Parnham Advisory Services
Hankelstrasse 43
D-53125 Bonn
Germany

A CIP catalogue record for this book is available from the Library of Congress, Washington, D.C., USA

Deutsche Bibliothek Cataloging-in-Publication Data

Non-opioids in pain management : Vancouver, Canada, August 19, 1996 / ed.: M. J. Parnham. – Basel ; Boston ; Berlin : Birkhäuser, 1997
ISBN 978-3-7643-5700-9   ISBN 978-3-0348-8904-9 (eBook)
DOI 10.1007/978-3-0348-8904-9
NE: Parnham, Michael J. [Hrsg.]

1997 Springer Basel AG
Originally published by Birkhäuser Verlag Basel, Switzerland in 1997
Printed on acid-free paper produced from chlorine-free pulp. TCF ∞

9 8 7 6 5 4 3 2 1

Contents

Preface 7

Introductory Remarks 9
K. A. Lehmann

Dipyrone in Pain Management 13
K. A. Lehmann

Treatment of Postoperative Pain Without Opioids 27
N. Rawal

Non-Opioid Analgesics in Cancer Pain Relief 37
S.A. Schug

Comparative Safety of Non-Opioid Analgesics 47
C. Martinez

Preface

There is no ideal analgesic and the most potent drug is not always the best because of its side-effects. Non-opioid analgesics, including the non-steroidal anti-inflammatory drugs and the non-narcotic analgesics, play an important role in the relief of a wide spectrum of painful conditions, though they vary in efficacy and safety. This book reviews the role which non-opioid analgesics play in the relief of pain, particularly with regard to postoperative and cancer pain. Emphasis is placed on the clinical indications for the non-acidic analgesic, dipyrone, and its relative safety in comparison to other non-opioid anlgesics.

Michael J. Parnham

Introductory remarks

Klaus A. Lehmann,
Department of Anaesthesiology
and Operative Intensive Care,
University of Cologne,
Josef-Stelzmann-Str. 9,
D-50924 Cologne, Germany

Opioids are considered to be the most potent analgesics for the management of acute and chronic pain. Much progress has been achieved with respect to their general availability in most countries, and health care personnel have been encouraged to use these drugs more generously in a variety of pain syndromes, including post-operative or cancer pain. The introduction of new techniques such as Patient-Controlled Analgesia (PCA) or guidelines such as the WHO ladder concept for cancer pain mangement have considerably increased our knowledge of their benefits and problems.

Opioid side-effects, including respiratory depression, sedation or constipation are typically dose-related. Attempts to reduce opioid dosages are therefore justified whenever possible. One of the easiest ways is to take advantage of combination with the well proven non-opioid analgesics. Several classes of non-opioid analgesic drugs are available including numerous non-steroidal anti-inflammatory drugs (NSAIDs) with their prominent antiinflammatory effects, and the antipyretic analgesics such as paracetamol or dipyrone.

Unlike opioids, which preferentially inhibit the synaptic transmission of nociceptive stimuli in the spinal cord and the brain, the antipyretic-antiinflammatory analgesics mainly increase nociceptor thresholds by inhibiting the enzyme cyclooxygenase, thus reducing the concentration of nociceptive mediators and neurotransmitters both peripherally and centrally.

Non-opioids have a long history as analgesics in inflammation, headache or trauma. If adequately used, they are effective for the management of late post-operative and early cancer pain, and particularly useful in drug combinations.

Dipyrone (metamizol, Novalgin") is a classical antipyretic analgesic of the pyrazolone class. Though not available everywhere it is marketed in more than 100 countries throughout the world. It was first launched in Germany in 1921 and was used widely as an over-the-counter analgesic.

Dipyrone has a similar analgesic efficacy to that of NSAIDs and tramadol probably due to an action on the spinal cord [1], but like para-cetamol, it has weak cyclo-oxygenase inhibitory activity. Consequently, unlike the NSAIDs, it has no relevant anti-inflammatory activity, but also little gastrointestinal irritant capacity. As described by Dr. Martinez in this volume, dipyrone is not associated with any mortality due to upper gastrointestinal bleeding.

A further unique characteristic of this drug is its intrinsic spasmolytic activity [2]. This makes dipyrone particularly useful in the treatment of renal and biliary colic pain.

Following reports in the late 1970´s which linked the use of dipyrone to cases of agranulocytosis, the drug was withdrawn in the United States and Sweden and changed to a prescription only analgesic in Germany. Extensive epidemiological studies since then have shown that the risk of agranulocytosis is very low [3]. In fact, the incidence of agranulocytosis is similar in countries in which dipyrone is marketed and those where it is not (Table 1) [4].

Table 1:
Drug-induced agranulocytosis, a rare event.

Period	Area	Dipyrone marketed	Cases/million people/year	Deaths/million people/year
1967–1968	Finland	+	10	N.A.
1966–1970	Sweden	+	2.5	0.8
1973–1978	Stockholm	±	9	1
1958–1984	Denmark	+	N.A.	0.4
1980–1984	various	+	6.2	0.5
1980–1985	USA	–	7.2	N.A.

Modified from ref. [4]. N.A. = not available

In view of the newer clinical data on dipyrone, the drug was reintroduced to the market in Sweden in 1995. Used with care and given slowly by intra-venous infusion, dipyrone is a valuable analgesic particularly for patients with colic pain and those at risk for gastric or renal complications. Because it is available for oral, intravenous or rectal administration, dipyrone plays an important role in pain management.

This book contains the proceedings of a symposium held at the 8th World Congress on Pain in Vancouver, Canada, to review the current knowledge on the use of non-opioids such as dipyrone in the treatment of post-operative and cancer pain.

References

1. Brune, K., The mode of action of non-acidic analgesics. In: Gerber, W.D., Nappi, G. (Eds.) Update of Non-Narcotic Analgesic Research. Birkhäuser, Basel, pp. 15–19 (1993).
2. Schroth, H.-J., Direct antispasmodic effect of metamizol on the smooth muscle of the efferent urinary and biliary tracts. Therapiewoche *39*, 1522–1525 (1989).
3. Kaufman, D.W., Kelly. J.P., Levy, M. and Shapiro, S., The Drug Etiology of Agranulocytosis and Aplastic Anemia. Oxford University Press, New York (1991).
4. Heimpel, H., Arzneimittelinduzierte Agranulozytose. Arzneimitteltherapie *12*, 101–107 (1994).

Dipyrone in pain management

Klaus A. Lehmann,
Department of Anesthesiology and Operative Care,
University of Cologne, Josef-Stelzmann-Straße 9,
D-50924 Cologne, Germany

Introduction

In view of its long history, it is not surprising that dipyrone (metamizole) has been used for the relief of pain of a wide variety of different causes. In many countries, especially in Germany, dipyrone or Novalgin® is almost a household name. In common with the other non-acidic, non-opioid analgesic paracetamol, past use often outstripped the clinical documentation of efficacy. However, publications on many randomized, double-blind controlled studies are now available in which dipyrone has been investigated in comparison to paracetamol or opioids for mild to moderate pain. Some of these studies are reviewed here to demonstrate the variety of painful conditions in which dipyrone has been shown to be effective, and more are available in the literature [1–9].

Post-operative pain

Dipyrone vs. paracetamol

Dipyrone is commonly used for the treatment of acute, post-operative pain. As long ago as 1980, in a double-blind comparative study of a single oral dose of 1 g dipyrone, 1 g paracetamol or placebo in 264 patients with severe post-episiotomy pain, dipyrone proved to be significantly more effective than paracetamol [10]. The results of this study (Fig. 1) have since been confirmed in different post-operative conditions in which dipyrone has been found to be consistently more effective than paracetamol [6, 11]. Other studies have demonstrated at least equipotency of both drugs [12].

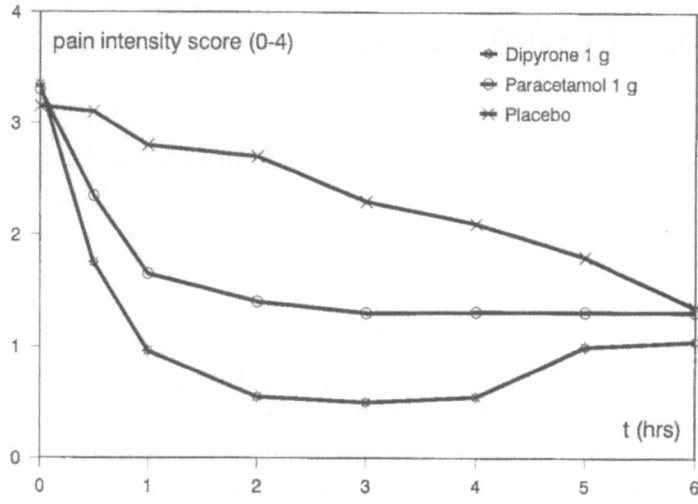

Fig. 1:
Mean pain scores after administration of a single oral dose of 1 g dipyrone (D), 1 g paracetamol (P) or placebo to 264 patients with severe post-episiotomy pain [6]. Both active treatments were significantly more effective than placebo.

Dipyrone vs. NSAIDs

Another commonly used analgesic is the non-steroidal anti-inflammatory drug (NSAID) aspirin. Dipyrone has also proved to be more effective than aspirin in the treatment of acute post-operative pain. For instance, in 254 patients with pain following repositioning of fractures due to trauma, a double-blind, placebo-controlled study revealed that oral 500 mg dipyrone provided greater pain relief than did oral 500 mg aspirin [13]. Similar findings were reported in other studies [6, 14, 15].

In a recent randomized, double-blind comparative study including 97 patients, 30 mg ketorolac, administered intramuscularly (i.m.), was compared with 2.5 g dipyrone, given by the same route [16]. The authors assessed the percentage of patients who were satisfied with the treatment in each group. Overall there was no difference between the therapy with either analgesic, and patients in both groups were equally satisfied with their treatment. Consequently, on parenteral administration the efficacy of this analgesic seems to be comparable to that of the NSAID, ketorolac. Comparable results were reported by Fernandez-Sabate et al. [17].

However, like all NSAIDs, which are inhibitors of cyclo-oxygenase and the synthesis of prostaglandins, ketorolac administration is associated with a greater risk of gastric and renal side-effects. For this reason dipyrone is generally preferred to NSAIDs for patients at risk of gastrointestinal or renal complications [18].

Dipyrone vs. opioids for mild to moderate pain

Because of its good analgesic efficacy and relatively low incidence of side-effects, dipyrone has also been shown to compare well with weak opioids for mild to moderate pain in the post-operative situation. One of the earliest randomized, double-blind studies was a comparative investigation of 2.5 g dipyrone and 100 mg pethidine given intravenously (i.v.) to 100 patients following laparoscopy [19, 20]. The course of pain relief was similar for both analgesics but dipyrone was better tolerated because of the higher incidence of nausea and vomiting in the patients on the opioid. For this reason, most patients in this study preferred dipyrone, which was later confirmed in a non-controlled trial [21].

Similar findings were made in a recent observer-blind multicentre study in which 2.5 g dipyrone was compared with 100 mg tramadol, both given i.v. [22]. Once again efficacy was similar, but the adverse events to tramadol were more pronounced than those to dipyrone. In experimental pain, in which oral 50–100 mg tramadol and 0.5–1 g dipyrone were compared, the tramadol:dipyrone analgesic equipotency ratio was estimated to be around 23:1 [23].

Dipyrone and the weak opioid tilidine, both administered orally to children suffering from traumatic pain, were found to be comparably effective in a randomised, double-blind comparison [24]. On the basis of data such as these, it is surprising that dipyrone, which is effective and well accepted by the patients, is not more widely used.

Currently, dipyrone is the only non-opioid analgesic which is available for administration intravenously as patient-controlled analgesia (PCA). In our institute, comparative data have been collected on groups of 40 patients each who underwent elective abdominal or orthopaedic surgery and were treated with PCA for about 24 h after the end of anaesthesia. The data obtained on dipyrone and various opioid drugs are shown in Table 1.

Though not as potent as the opioids, dipyrone approaches tramadol and pethidine in efficacy [25]. Only a few other studies, mostly uncontrolled, have been carried out using dipyrone for PCA [26–29].

Table 1:
Equipotency studies on analgesics administered as PCA to patients with severe pain following abdominal or urological surgery (data from [25]).

Analgesic	Demand dose (µg)	Maximum hourly dose (mg/h)	Consumption		Retrospective pain score (0–5)	Relative equipotent dose (product)
			(µg/kg/h)	(mg/70 kg/ day)		
Sufentanil[a]	6	0.04	0.10	0.2	1.85	0.004
Fentanyl	34	0.25	0.46	0.8	1.07	0.01
Buprenorphine	40	0.32	0.63	1.1	1.57	0.02
Alfentanil	212	1.5	4.96	8.3	1.37	0.15
Hydromorphone	566	2.94	6.60	11.1	2.25	0.33
1-Methadone	1145	5.95	14.20	23.9	1.60	0.50
Piritramide	1990	15.0	30.44	51.1	1.42	0.96
Morphine	1920	14.8	29.60	49.7	1.52	1
Nalbuphine	3846	28.5	117.52	197.4	1.82	4.75
Pentazocine	7980	60.0	135.57	227.8	1.60	4.82
Nefopam	3846	28.5	132.75	223.0	2.90	8.56
Pethidine	9615	100.0	175.10	294.2	2.22	8.63
Tramadol	9615	100.0	203.12	341.2	2.27	10.24
Dipyrone	50000	500.0	1804.21	3031	3.02	121.09

The table shows the dose parameters, mean analgesic consumption, and a retrospective pain score (0: no pain at all; 5: discontinued because of lack of efficacy). Relative equipotencies were calculated from the product of the 24 h consumption and the retrospective pain score, and are related to morphine as 1. All values are arithmetic means.
[a] 40 gynaecology patients treated with sufentanil

Dipyrone in combination with opioids

The majority of acutely painful surgical conditions in Germany are treated intravenously with a combination (in 500 ml) of 2.5–5.0 g dipyrone, 300–400 mg tramadol and haloperidol or droperidol to prevent emesis [30, 31]. This infusion mixture is an inexpensive and broadly applicable regimen which is widely accepted [32], although only one controlled study has been published [33]. Both tramadol and dipyrone are non-restricted drugs, which explains the popularity of the mixture on general wards. Where this regimen is unsuitable in individual patients, due to insufficient analgesia and/or side effects of tramadol, it is possible to switch to more effective, but also more expensive techniques such as patient-controlled-analgesia (PCA) using more potent opioids.

There are several reports in the literature that dipyrone is very useful in reducing the overall requirement for postoperative opioids. A very recent randomized, double-blind study on the administration of 1 g dipyrone 3 times every 24 h to reduce the requirement for buprenorphine in PCA was carried out in 100 patients with severe pain following abdominal or urological surgery [34]. As shown in Fig. 2, depending on the type of surgery performed, there was a significant reduction by dipyrone of the dose of buprenorphine required. In soft-tissue surgery, dipyrone did not provide any additional analgesic benefit. A follow-up study by the same group obtained even better results by administering as PCA a combination of dipyrone and diclofenac together with buprenorphine [35]. Other drug-interaction studies using dipyrone and various opioids for PCA are available in the literature and reach comparable conclusions [36, 37].

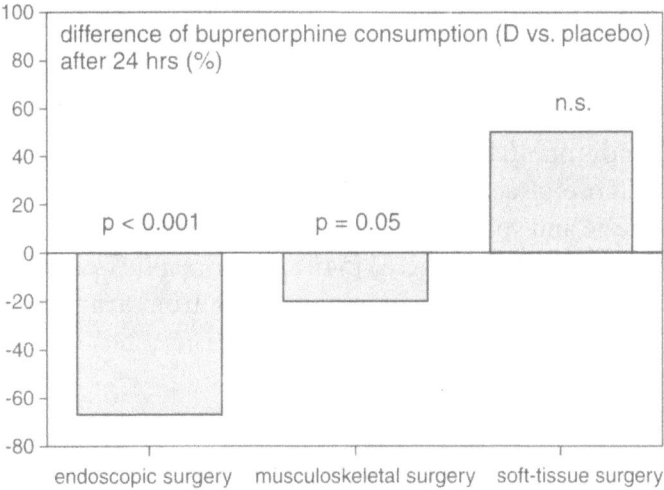

Fig. 2:
Reduction of the requirement for buprenorphine (B) in PCA by 1 g dipyrone (D) given 3 times every 24 h [34] to 100 patients with postoperative pain.

Dipyrone can therefore be recommended as a single analgesic for weak to moderate postoperative or traumatic pain management and is particularly useful in combination with an opioid for more severe pain, as long as no strong anti-inflammatory effects are required.

Dental pain

Following positive data from volunteer studies on experimental tooth pulp pain [23, 38, 39], several investigations provided promising clinical results in patients suffering from tooth extraction pain [6, 10, 40]. Obviously, more controlled studies are required for this pain situation.

Spastic pain

The intrinsic spasmolytic properties of dipyrone make it particularly suited to the treatment of spastic or colic pain [41–46]. Many randomized, double-blind studies have been carried out in this indication, predominantly with dipyrone, diclofenac, tramadol or pethidine [47–53]. Dipyrone tends to be superior to tramadol and pethidine in pain relief and comparable to NSAIDs. However, patients usually prefer dipyrone because of the higher incidence of gastrointestinal side-effects among the NSAIDs.

N-Butylscopolamine, a hyoscine derivative, is a spasmolytic agent which is often used in the treatment of colic pain. In a recent randomised double-blind study on 104 patients with renal colic, 2.5 g dipyrone i.v. proved to be a more effective analgesic in this condition, because of its combined analgesic and spasmolytic effects, than either 100 mg tramadol or 20 mg N-butylscopolamine (Fig. 3) [54]. Similar results were obtained in 96 renal patients [55] and in 74 patients suffering from acute biliary colic pain [56].

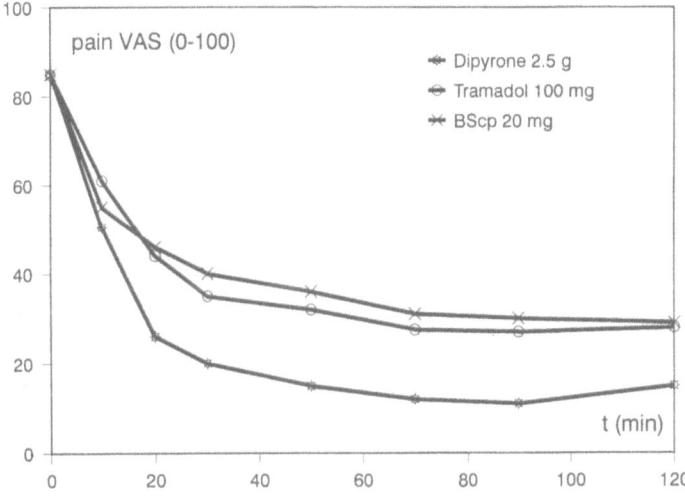

Fig. 3:
Comparative efficacy of dipyrone, tramadol and N-butylscopolamine (BScp) in the treatment
of 104 patients with acute renal colic pain [54].

Sciatic pain

The number of patients who suffer from sciatic pain is relatively large.
NSAIDs are commonly used for the treatment of this type of pain. In a
randomised observer-blind study of 260 patients, 2.5 g dipyrone i.m. has
been shown to be at least as effective in the relief of sciatic pain as 75 mg
diclofenac [57]. Dipyrone, however, has a longer duration of action, particularly on the second day of treatment, and was better tolerated than diclofenac (Fig. 4). Less rescue medication was required with dipyrone than
with diclofenac on the second day.

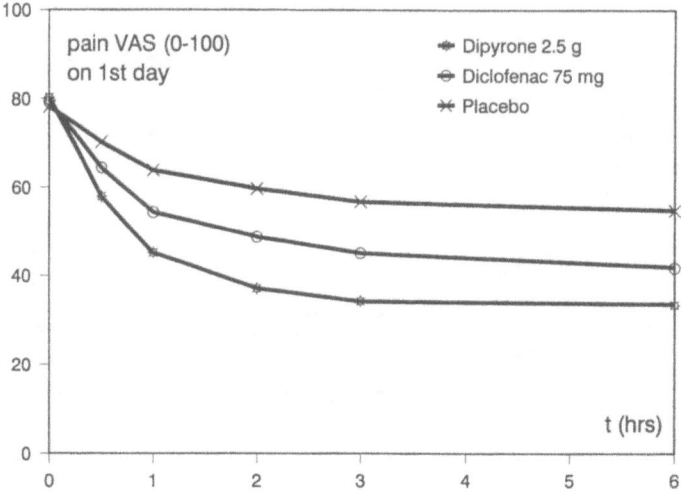

Fig. 4.
Comparison of the efficacy of intramuscular dipyrone and diclofenac in the treatment of 261 patients with acute lumbago or sciatic pain [57].

Cancer pain

The WHO analgesic ladder is widely used as the basis for the drug therapy of cancer pain. Non-opioid analgesics are recommended as single agents on the first step of the ladder and as adjuvants on the later rungs. Within our institution, dipyrone is often used as the non-opioid analgesic of first choice. In a retrospective study of more than 1000 cancer patients [58], we found that NSAIDs were used in about 40% of cases, often as single analgesics on step I, but the non-acidic analgesics, dipyrone and paracetamol, were used more frequently than NSAIDs, particularly at steps II and III (Fig. 5). Dipyrone alone, at a mean dose of 4.6 g per day, was used in 40% of cases and paracetamol alone in 6% of cases. This preference is explained by the fact that dipyrone and paracetamol have a lower incidence of side-effects than do the NSAIDs. Similar results which are also valid in children and adolescents were obtained by other researchers [59–61].

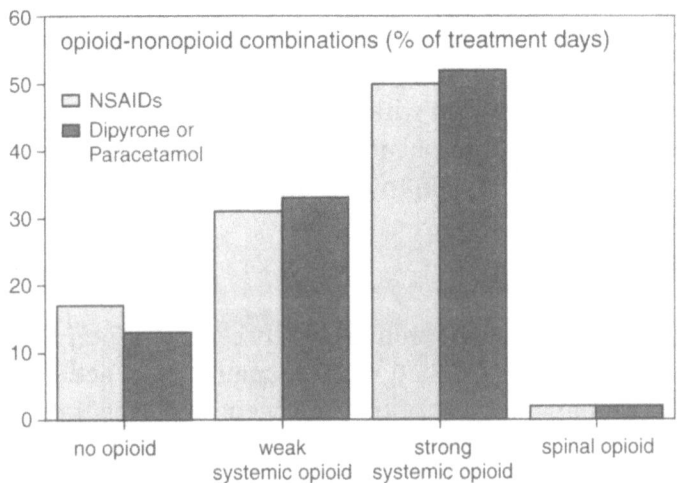

Fig. 5:
The use of non-opioid analgesics in the management of cancer pain according to the WHO concept [58]. Data were obtained from a retrospective study of 1070 cancer pain patients who received treatment for a total of 55,285 days. Non-opioids alone were used for 12.6% of the time and in combination with opioids for 73.3% of the time.

Conclusions

In addition to the many decades of practical experience with dipyrone, particularly in Germany, randomized, double-blind clinical trials have confirmed the efficacy of this non-opioid analgesic in a variety of painful conditions. In post-operative pain, dipyrone is as effective as and better tolerated than NSAIDs and is the only non-opioid analgesic which can be used for PCA, alone or in combination with opioids. Due to its additional, intrinsic spasmolytic activity, dipyrone has been found to be superior to tramadol, pethidine and N-butylscopolamine in the treatment of spastic pain, in which it has the advantage once again over NSAIDs of improved tolerability. This better tolerability gives dipyrone an edge over NSAIDs in the treatment of sciatic pain and as a co-analgesic in cancer pain, though its weak cyclo-oxygenase-inhibiting activity is a disadvantage for relief of inflammatory pain. In the view of the author, dipyrone offers valuable therapeutic options particularly for patients with smooth muscle pain, those who are at risk of gastric or renal intolerance, of postoperative bleeding or respiratory depression, and for patients who are at risk of cognitive dysfunctions. Although the literature contains enough data to justify such a conclusion, additional research with strictly controlled protocols will further elucidate the role of dipyrone in our pain armamentarium. Researchers all over the world are invited to gain their own experience.

Floor discussion

Asked whether dipyrone has a predominantly central or peripheral mechanism of action, Lehmann replied that the main site of action is central. Although it is a weak inhibitor of cyclo-oxygenase peripherally, dipyrone can easily enter the central nervous system where it can accumulate to inhibit central prostaglandin synthesis. This and probably other central actions, which are independent of opioid mechanisms, make a major contribution to the analgesic activity of dipyrone [62–69].

References

1. Alon, E., Biro, P., Himmelseher, S.: Zur Lage der Schmerzbehandlung durch Anästhesiologen in der Deutschschweiz. Eur. J. Pain 14, 91–96 (1993).
2. Brune, K., 100 Jahre Pyrazolone. Eine Bestandsaufnahme. Urban & Schwarzenberg, München Wien Baltimore (1985).
3. Bierbach, H., Die Behandlung akuter gastrointestinaler Schmerzen. Schmerz 7, 154–159 (1993).
4. Brune, K. (ed), New clinical and epidemiological data on dipyrone. Birkhäuser, Basel Boston Berlin (1993)
5. Cherny, N.I., Portenoy, R.K., Raber, M., Zenz, M., Medikamentöse Therapie von Tumorschmerzen. Teil 1: Eigenschaften von Nichtopioiden und Opioiden. Schmerz 8, 195–200 (1994).
6. Gerbert, W.D., Napp, G. (eds), Update on non-narcotic analgesic research. Birkhäuser, Basel Boston Berlin (1993)
7. Lehmann, K.A., On-Demand Analgesie: Neue Möglichkeiten zur Behandlung akuter Schmerzen. Arzneimittelforschung 34, 1108–1114 (1984).
8. Piepenbrock, S., Schäffer, J., Zenz, M., Analgesie bei Unfallverletzten. Dtsch. Ärztebl. 86, 236–238 (1989).
9. Thole, H., Tryba, M., Zenz, M., Postoperative Analgesie – systemische vs. regionale Schmerztherapie. Anaesth. Intensivmed. 212, 190–198 (1990).
10. Gómez-Jiménez, J., Franco-Patino, R., Chargoy-Vera, J. and Olivares-Sosa, R., Clinical efficacy of mild analgesics in pain following gynaecological or dental surgery: report on multicentre studies. Br. J. Clin. Pharmacol. 10, 355S–358S (1980).
11. Daftary, S.N., Mehta, A.C., Nanavati, M., A controlled comparison of dipyrone and paracetamol in post-episiotomy pain. Curr. Med. Res. Opin. 6, 614–618 (1980).

12. Farkas, J.C., Larrouturou, P., Morin, J.P., et al., Analgesic efficacy of an injectable acetaminophene versus a dipyrone plus pitofenone plus feniverinium associated after abdominal aortic repair. Curr. Ther. Res. 51, 19–27 (1992).

13. Mehta, S.D., A randomized double-blind placebo-controlled study of dipyrone and aspirin in post-operative orthopaedic patients. J. Int. Med. Res. 14, 63–66 (1986).

14. Blendinger, I., Eberlein, H.J., Comparison of intravenous acetylsalicylic acid and dipyrone in postoperative pain: an interim report. Br. J. Clin. Pharmacol. 10, 339S–341S (1980).

15. Murkherjee, S., Sood, S., A controlled evaluation of orally administered aspirin, dipyrone and placebo in patients with post-operative pain. Curr. Med. Res. Opin. 6, 619–623 (1980).

16. Ibarra-Ibarra, L.G., Cubillo, M.A., Silva-Adaya, A., Gonzales-Garcia, C.A., Comparative study of ketorolac and dipyrone in the treatment of postoperative pain. Proc. West. Pharmacol. Soc. 36, 133–135 (1993).

17. Fernandez-Sabate, A., Roca-Burniol, J., Roca-Barbera, A., Gonzalez-Caudevilla, B., Ketorolac, a new nonopioid analgesic, in a single-blind trial versus metamizol in orthopaedic surgery pain. Curr. Ther. Res. 49, 1016–1024 (1992).

18. Laporte, J.R., Carné, X., Vidal, X., Moreno, V., Juan, J., Upper gastrointestinal bleeding in relation to previous use of analgesics and non-steroidal anti-inflammatory drugs. Lancet 337, 85–89 (1991).

19. Patel, C.V., Koppikar, M.G., Patel, M.S., A double-blind comparison of parenteral dipyrone and pethidine in the treatment of post-operative pain. Curr. Med. Res. Opin. 6, 624–629 (1980).

20. Patel, C.V., Koppikar, M.G., Patel, M.S., Parulkar, G.B., Pinto Pereira, L.M., Management of pain after abdominal surgery: dipyrone compared with pethidine. Br. J. Clin. Pharmacol. 10, 351S–354S (1980).

21. Casali, R., Novelli, G.P., Bonetti, L., Comparison of dipyrone and pethidine in surgical pain. Anest. Rianim. 22, 143–154 (1981).

22. Stankov, G., Schmieder, G., Lechner, F.J., Schinzel, S., Observer-blind multicentre study with dipyrone versus tramadol in postoperative pain. Eur. J. Pain 16, 56–63 (1995).

23. Rohdewald, P., Granitzky, H.W., Neddermann, E., Comparison of the analgesic efficacy of metamizole and tramadol in experimental pain. Pharmacology 37, 209–207 (1988).

24. von Bülow, H., Die analgetische Wirkung von Tilidin im Vergleich zu Metamizol-Tropfen bei posttraumatischen Schmerzen im Kindesalter. Therapiewoche 38, 1232–1234 (1988).

25. Lehmann, K.A., Patient-controlled analgesia for the treatment of postoperative pain. Zentralbl. Chir. 120, 1–15 (1995).

26. Juhl, G., Der Infucommand. Ein PCA-Gerät mit pulsoxymetrischer Boluskontrolle. Anaesthesist 39, 236–239 (1990).

27. Rodriguez, M.J., de la Torre, M.R., Perez-Iraola, P., et al., Comparative study of tramadol versus NSAIDs as intravenous continuous infusion for managing postoperative pain. Curr. Ther. Res. 54, 375–383 (1993)

28. Torres, L.M., Collado, F., Almarcha, et al., Tratamiento del dolor postoperatorio con sistima de PCA intravenoso. Comparación entre morfina, metamizol y buprenorfina. Rev. Esp. Anestesiol. Reanim. 40, 181–184 (1993).

29. Ure, B.M., Neugebauer, E., Ullmann, K., Driever, R., Troidl, H., Patientenkontrollierte Analgesie (PCA) zur postoperativen Schmerztherapie. Eine prospektive Beobachtungsstudie zur Technologiebewertung im Stationsbetrieb. Chirurg 64, 802–808 (1993).

30. Dauber, A., Ure, B.M., Neugebauer, E., Schmitz, S., Troidl, H., Zur Inzidenz postoperativer Schmerzen auf chirurgischen Normalstationen. Ergebnisse unterschiedlicher Evaluierungsverfahren. Anaesthesist 42, 448–454 (1993).
31. Krümmer, H., Pfeiffer, H., Arbogast, R., Sprotte, G., Die kombinierte Infusionsanalgesie – ein alternatives Konzept zur postoperativen Schmerztherapie. Chirurg 57, 327–329 (1986).
32. Lehmann, K.A., Henn, C., Zur Lage der postoperativen Schmerztherapie in der Bundesrepublik Deutschland. Ergebnisse einer Repräsentativumfrage. Anaesthesist 36, 400–406 (1987).
33. Striebel, H.W., Hackenberger, J., Vergleich einer Tramadol-/Metamizol-Infusion mit der Kombination von Tramadol-Infusion plus Ibuprofen-Suppositorien zur postoperativen Schmerztherapie nach Hysterektomien. Anaesthesist 41, 354–360 (1992).
34. Steffen, P., Schuhmacher, I., Weichel, T., Georgieff, M., Seeling, W., Untersuchungen zum differenzierten Einsatz von Nichtopioiden zur postoperativen Analgesie. I. Quantifizierung des analgetischen Effektes von Metamizol mittels der patientenkontrollierten Analgesie. Anaesthesiol Intensivmed Notfallmed Schmerzther 31, 143–147 (1996).
35. Steffen, P., Drück, A., Krinn, et al., Untersuchungen zum differenzierten Einsatz von Nichtopioiden zur postoperativen Analgesie. II. Quantifizierung des analgetischen Effektes der Kombination von Metamizol plus Diclofenac mittels der patientenkontrollierten Analgesie. Anaesthesiol Intensivmed Notfallmed Schmerzther 31, 216–221 (1996).
36. Jage, J., Göb, J., Wagner, W., Henneberg, T., Lehmann, K.A., Postoperative Schmerztherapie mit Piritramid und Metamizol. Eine randomisierte Untersuchung an 120 abdominal-chirurgischen Patienten im Rahmen der intravenösen On-Demand Analgesie. Schmerz 4, 29–36 (1990).
37. Lehmann, K.A., Abu-Shibika, M., Horrichs-Haermeyer, G., Postoperative Schmerztherapie mit l-Methadon und Metamizol. Eine randomisierte Untersuchung im Rahmen der intravenösen On-Demand Analgesie. Anaesth Intensivther Notfallmed 25, 152–159 (1990).
38. Pöllmann, L., Über tageszeitliche Unterschiede der Wirksamkeit eines Analgetikums. Dtsch. Zahnaerztl. Z. 31, 812–814 (1976).
39. Rohdewald, P., Neddermann, E., Dosisabhängigkeit der analgetischen Wirkung von Metamizol. Anaesthesist 37, 150–155 (1988).
40. Altamash, M., Kalkhammer, R., Open clinical trial to determine the analgesic effects of metamizol and mefenamic acid after extraction of lower impacted wisdom tooth. Hoechst Internal Report (1989).
41. Laird, J.M.A., Cervero, F., Effects of metamizol on nociceptor responses to stimulation of the ureter and on reter mobility in anesthetised rats. Inflamm. Res. 45, 150–154 (1996).
42. Schroth, H.J., Steinsträßer, A., Berberich, R., Kloss, G., Motilität der ableitenden Harnwege. Änderung des Ausscheidungsphase im Nierensequenzszintigramm unter der Wirkung von Metamizol – ein Parameter zur Beurteilung. MMW 127, 227–228 (1985).
43. Schroth, H.J., Garth, H., Rupp, S., Steinsträßer, A., Wirkung von Metamizol auf die Harnwegs-Motilität. Eine quantitative Analyse der Ausscheidungsphase der Nierensequenz-Szintigraphie. Fortschr. Med. 104, 378–382 (1986).
44. Schroth, H.J., Garth, H., Rupp, S., Oberhausen, E., Wirkung von Metamizol auf die Kontraktilität der Gallenblase. Fortschr. Med. 105. 136–138 (1987).

45. Schroth, H.J., Direct antispasmodic effect of metamiozol on the smooth muscle of the efferent urinary and biliary tracts. Therapiewoche 39, 1522–1525 (1989).
46. Stähler, G., Die Harnleiterkolik. Internist 30, 110–113 (1989).
47. Arnau, J.M., Cami, J., Garcia-Alonso, F., Laporte, J.R., Palop, R., Comparative study of the efficacy of dipyrone, diclofenac sodium and pethidine in acute renal colic. Eur. J. Clin. Pharmacol. 40, 543–546 (1991).
48. Haag Molkenteller, C., Results of clinical trials with dipyrone (metamizol) in acute postoperative pain and colicky pain. Klin. Pharmakol. Akt. 7, 33–40 (1996)
49. Miralles, R., Cami, J., Guitiérrez, J., et al., Diclofenac versus dipyrone in acute renal colic: a double-blind controlled trial. Eur. J. Pharmacol. 33, 527–528 (1987).
50. Lehtonen, T., Kellokumpu, I., Permi, I., Sarsila, O., Intravenous indomethacin in the treatment of ureteric colic. A clinical multicentre study with pethidine and metamizol as the control preparations. Ann. Clin. Res. 15, 197–199 (1983).
51. Muriel, C., Ortiz, P., and the Cooperative Group: Efficacy of two different intramuscular doses of dipyrone in acute renal colic. Meth. Find. Exp. Clin. Pharmacol. 15, 465–469 (1993).
52. Muriel-Villoria, C., Zungri-Telo, E., Diaz-Curiel, M., et al., Comparison of the onset and duration of dipyrone, 1 or 2 g, by the intramuscular or intravenous route, in acute renal colic. Eur. J. Clin. Pharmacol. 48, 103–107 (1995).
53. Primus, G., Pummer, K., Vucsina, F., Meindl, N., Tramadol versus Metimazol zur Schmerzausschaltung bei Ureterkolik, Urologe (A) 28, 103–105 (1989).
54. Stankov, G., Schmieder, G., Zerle, G., Schinzel, S., Brune, K., Double-blind study with dipyrone versus tramadol and butylscopolamine in acute renal colic pain. World K. Urol. 12, 155–161 (1993).
55. Lloret, J., Munoz, J., Monmany, J., et al., Treatment of renal colic with dipyrone. A double-blind comparison trial with hyoscine alone or combined with dipyrone. Curr. Ther. Res. 42, 1119–1128 (1987).
56. Schmieder, G., Stankov, G., Zerle, G., Schinzel S., Brune, K., Observer-blind study with metamizol versus tramadol and butylscopolamine in acute biliary colic pain. Arzneimittelforschung 43, 1216–1221 (1993).
57. Babej-Dölle, R., Freytag, S., Eckmeyer, J., et al., Parenteral dipyrone versus diclofenac and placebo in patients with acute lumbago or sciatic pain: randomised observer-blind multicenter study. Int. J. Clin. Pharmacol. Ther. 32, 204–209 (1994).
58. Grond S., Zech, D., Schug, S.A., Lynch, J., Lehmann, K.A., The importance of non-opioid analgesics for cancer pain relief according to the guidelines of the World Health Organization. Int. J. Clin. Pharmacol. Res. 11, 253–260 (1991).
59. Rodriguez, M., Barutell, C., Rull, et al., Efficacy and tolerance of oral dipyrone versus oral morphine for cancer pain. Eur. J. Cancer 30, 584–587 (1994).
60. Schlunk, T., Friess, D., Winterhalder, D., Kontinuierliche subakute Schmerztherapie mit peripher und zentral wirkenden Analgetika. Med. Welt 45, 553–558 (1994).
61. Sittl, R., Richter, R., Tumorschmerztherapie bei Kindern und Jugendlichen mit Morphin. Anaesthesist 40, 96–99 (1991).
62. Brune, K., Alpermann, H., Non-acidic pyrazoles: inhibition of prostaglandin production, carrageenan oedema and yeast fever. Agents Actions 13, 360–363 (1983).
63. Carlsson, K.H., Helmreich, J., Jurna, I., Activation of inhibition from the periaqueductal grey matter mediates central analgesic effects of metamizol (dipyrone). Pain 27, 373–390 (1986)
64. Carlsson, K.H., Helmreich, J., Jurna, I., Comparison of central antinociceptive and analgesic effects of the pyrazolone derivatives, metamizol (dipyrone) and amiphenazone («Pyramidone»). Schmerz-Pain-Douleur 7, 93–100 (1986).

65. Carlsson, K.H., Jurna, I., The role of descending inhibition in the antinociceptive effects of the pyrazolone derivatives, metamizol (dipyrone) and amiphenazone («Pyramidone»)- Naunyn-Schmiedebergs Arch. Pharmacol. 335, 154–159 (1987).
66. Carlsson, K.H., Monzel, W., Jurna, I., Depression by morphine and the non-opioid analgesic agents, metamizol (dipyrone), lysine acetylsalicylate, and paracetamol, of activity in rat thalamus neurones evoked by electrical stimulation of nociceptive afferents. Pain 32, 313–326 (1988).
67. Ferreira, S.H., The mode of action of peripheral analgesics: blockade of inflammatory hyperalgesia. Schmerz-Pain-Douleur 9, 103–109 (1988).
68. Neugebauer, V., Schaible, H.G., He, X., et al., Electrophysiological evidence for a spinal antinociceptive action of dipyrone. Agents Actions 41, 62–70 (1994).
69. Weithmann, K.U., Alpermann, H.G., Biochemical and pharmacological effects of dipyrone and ist metabolites in model systems related to arachidonic acid cascade. Arzneimittelforschung 35, 947–952 (1985).

Treatment of postoperative pain without opioids

Narinder Rawal,
Department of Anesthesiology and Intensive Care,
Örebro Medical Center Hospital,
S-701 85 Örebro, Sweden

Introduction

In spite of unprecedented interest in postoperative pain and its manage-ment, most patients undergoing surgery do not receive adequate analgesia on surgical wards. In a recent survey of 300 hospitals and 500 households in the United States, it was found that about 80% of patients still have pain after surgery [1], despite the availability of a variety of guidelines on the effective management of pain (Table 1).

Table 1:
Results of a survey of post-operative pain management in the United States [1].

Hospitals surveyed:	300
Households surveyed:	500
Hospitals with acute pain management programmes:	42% (+ 13% planned)
Adults (households) having undergone surgery in last 5 years:	27%
Patients reporting pain after surgery:	77%
Patients with pain after first analgesic dose:	71%
Patients experiencing side-effects:	23%
Patients considering pain after surgery to be necessary:	77%
Patients prefering non-opioid to opioid after surgery:	71%

In a recent Swedish survey of over 1000 day surgery patients, almost every third patient undergoing surgery had post-operative pain at home [2]. The most common technique for providing postoperative analgesia remains the use of i.m. opioids prescribed by surgeons and administered by ward nurses on an as-needed basis. The inadequacies of this method of pain management are well recognized [3–5]. It is increasingly clear that if post-operative analgesia is to be improved on surgical wards, techniques such as PCA, epidural analgesia and peripheral nerve blocks have to be introduced on a routine basis. These techniques provide superior analgesia in comparison to i.m. opioids but have their own risks and therefore require special monitoring. Traditional methods of analgesia are not risk-free either but the risks have rarely been quantified. While better postoperative pain is relatively easily achieved, there has to be a balance between acceptable risk, perceived benefit and cost-effectiveness. Without an effective organization of postoperative pain services, pain management on surgical wards will remain unsatisfactory [6]. Furthermore, quality assurance measures such as frequent recording of pain intensity and treatment efficacy can no longer be ignored. The recent explosion of interest in Patient-Controlled Analgesia (PCA), nonsteroidal anti-inflammatory drugs (NSAIDs) and other non-opioids, intraspinal opioids, regional analgesia techniques and organization of Acute Pain Services is a direct response to this realization [7].

The importance of patient selection by the anesthesiologist for different analgesic therapies cannot be overemphasized; this has major implications for cost-effectiveness and postoperative morbidity. It should be noted that sophisticated analgesia techniques such as epidural administration and PCA are neither necessary nor realistic for most patients. The majority of surgical patients are ASA class 1 or 2 and most surgical procedures are such that early restoration of respiratory function or early ambulation are not a major problem. Such patients can be managed adequately by appropriate use of peripherally acting analgesics such as NSAIDs and/ or centrally acting systemic opioids.

Use of non-opioids for postoperative pain

Aspirin, paracetamol and NSAIDs are the main non-opioid analgesics for treating mild to moderate postoperative pain. Dipyrone, a non-opioid analgesic which has been marketed worldwide since 1922, was reintroduced in Sweden in 1995 for postoperative pain. These drugs are used as sole analgesics or given in combination with other analgesic drugs such as opioids or with analgesic techniques such as peripheral nerve blocks. There is a «ceiling effect» to the analgesia with these drugs in that further increases in dose do not result in additional pain relief. Non-opioids may be particularly suitable in procedures involving musculoskeletal, post-traumatic and inflammatory pain in which prostaglandins are known to be pathogenetically involved [8,9]. When used as a component of «multimodal balanced analgesia» such drugs have resulted in 20–40% reduction in opioid requirement [10]. This can be expected to reduce opioid related morbidity. However, there is no convincing evidence so far that this «opioid sparing» effect results in a reduced risk of adverse effects. Moreover, balanced analgesia with multiple analgesics may lead to addititve effects or to synergism of the drugs. The latter is obviously desirable with regard to analgesic efficacy as long as adverse effects are also not enhanced. A further complication is that there are no clear guidelines on the optimal routes of administration for balanced analgesia and clearly further studies are required in this area.

It is debatable whether NSAIDs provide any advantage over simple analgesics, such as paracetamol or dipyrone in the treatment of post-operative pain, not only in terms of efficacy but also in relation to side-effects. In a recent double-blind comparative study of paracetamol and ketorolac, pain relief with both compounds was similar, but blood loss was significantly higher after ketorolac. In addition, the treatment with the NSAID was more expensive and the cost of treating «nuisance bleeding» raises the expense even further [11].

The ever increasing number of outpatient surgeries creates a demand upon anesthesiologists to provide the essential features of rapid outpatient recovery – the four A's of alertness, analgesia, alimentation and ambulation. These patients must be capable of entering a medically unsupervised environment without adverse effects such as severe pain, nausea, vomiting and sedation. Pain may be a major cause of postoperative nausea and vomiting. However, treatment of pain by i.m. opioids is also associated with nausea, vomiting and sedation which may result in many patients having to remain in hospital, thus defeating the objective of day-stay planning. Oral or rectal administration of potent NSAIDs for prevention and management of postoperative pain in day-care patients appears to be gaining increasing acceptance.

Non-opioids in pre-emptive analgesia

Non-opioid analgesics have also been used for «pre-emptive analgesia» in several studies [12]. The concept of pre-emptive analgesia, that pretreatment can prevent pain after surgery or trauma, is based on neurophysiological animal experimental data. There is convincing evidence that acute afferent barrages associated with tissue trauma will generate changes in spinal sensory processing that lead to a hyperalgesic state which may account for the postsurgical pain state [13]. Several clinical studies have evaluated possible pre-emptive analgesic effects by preoperative or intraoperative treatment using regional or local anesthesia techniques, systemic or epidural opioids [14–16], NSAIDs or paracetamol [17–19].

Although some clinical studies have duplicated the impressive results from animal studies, the hypothesis that pretreatment before surgery can significantly reduce postoperative pain and hyperalgesia has generally been a disappointment. Nevertheless, the pre-emptive analgesia debate has focused attention on the importance of using analgesia-based pre- and intraoperative anesthesia techniques. Surgical stimulation of pain processes, unlike the experimental models, persists for periods that outlast the effect of treatment [20–21]. Ongoing nociceptive impulse barrage of the spinal cord neurons from the surgical wound will continue long after the effect of any pre-treatment has worn off. It would appear, therefore, that pre-emptive analgesia will be clinically meaningful only when started before surgery and continued as long as nociceptors are stimulated in the wound area. At our institution every patient who undergoes surgery (about 20,000 patients a year) receives 1 g paracetamol 4 times a day as «base medication». This treatment begins preoperatively and continues until the patient is completely pain-free for at least 6–8 hours, children receive 15–20 mg/kg orally or rectally (Table 2).

Table 2:
Standard orders for use of analgesics on surgical wards (Örebro Medical Centre Hospital, Sweden) [from 5]

---

1. Record pain intensity (on bedside flow sheet) every 3 h. VAS recording may be terminated only when VAS is 3 or less without treatment on 3 consecutive measurements.
2. Unless contraindicated (e.g. liver disease) give every adult 1 g paracetamol rectally (suppository) 4–6 times a day as base analgesic medication until VAS recording is terminated. For children 15–20 mg/kg rectally.
3. In addition, morphine 7.5–10 mg when VAS > 3 (reduce doses by 25–50% in elderly and very sick patients). Re-check and record VAS about 45 min after morphine injection. If VAS > 3 give additional morphine (50% of initial dose).
4. Contact APN or section anesthesiologists Dr. .... if VAS > after second dose. After working hours, contact the anesthesiologist on-call.

Regional techniques for postoperative analgesia

The use of parenteral opioids for treating postoperative pain is associated with several adverse effects such as sedation, respiratory depression, nausea and depression of gastrointestinal function. By avoiding opioids, regional anesthetic techniques provide excellent analgesia in an alert, cooperative patient untroubled by nausea.

Regional anesthesia techniques are among the most effective and versatile means for providing relief of acute pain (Fig. 1). Single injection techniques may be useful after outpatient and minor surgery. In the hospitalized patient who has undergone a more extensive surgical procedure, a catheter (continuous) technique is preferable. Wound infiltration is perhaps the simplest method for providing wound analgesia but is all too fre-

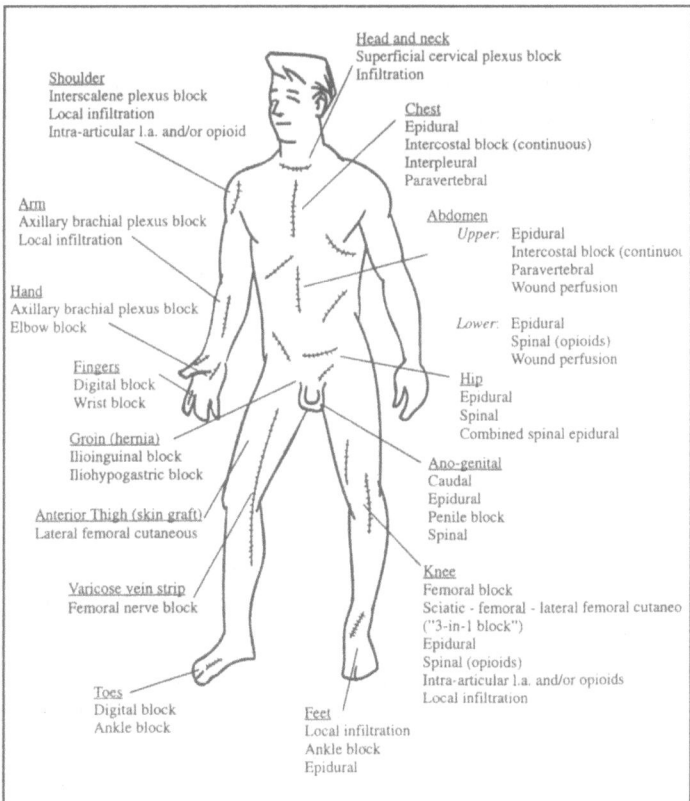

Fig. 1:
Regional anaesthetic techniques available for the day-care patient

quently neglected. At our institution, patients routinely receive infiltration of the wound with a local anaesthetic before closure of the surgical wound.

Any peripheral nerve block (brachial plexus, sciatic, femoral, intercostal) performed with a long-acting local anesthetic such as bupivacaine provides analgesia which may last up to 6–8 h. Wrist, ankle and elbow blocks are easy to perform. Equally simple and effective are ilioinguinal and iliohypogastric blocks following hemiography and intercostal block following upper abdominal or thoracic surgery. In general, appropriate blocks exist for almost all areas of the body. Catheter techniques have been described for several peripheral blocks [13]. Catheters can be introduced into the brachial plexus, using a three-in-one block, in the femoral nerve lumbar plexus or intercostal space. Although continuous peripheral nerve blocks by the catheter technique are easy to perform, cost effective and safe, and provide excellent analgesia of long duration, they remain underused for postoperative pain management.

Of all the techniques available for postoperative pain relief none provides greater versatility than epidural block with catheter technique. Analgesia can be provided from upper chest to toes. Epidural block is increasingly a part of the anesthetic technique; the catheter can be used to extend the block during the postoperative period. Local anesthetics or opioids or a combination of these drugs will provide excellent postoperative analgesia. Caudal anesthesia is probably the commonest regional anesthetic technique for surgery below the umbilicus and for postoperative analgesia in children. It is generally considered to be a simple, safe and effective block.

Conclusion

A variety of simple ways exist for opioid-sparing in post-operative pain relief. These include pre-operative information, good premedication, «base medication» with a simple analgesic such as paracetamol or perhaps dipyrone, wound infiltration and peripheral nerve block. In our institution, patients receive extensive pre-operative information about pain assessment by visual analogue scale (VAS) and about available pain management techniques and the rationale underlying their use. This is reinforced by information brochures and wall posters (Fig. 2) which inform patients about the importance of effective postoperative pain relief. Frequent assessment of pain intensity by VAS is performed and patients are told that every effort will be made to keep their VAS at or below 3 on the 10 grade scale. Here the use of non-opioid analgesics is playing an increasingly important role.

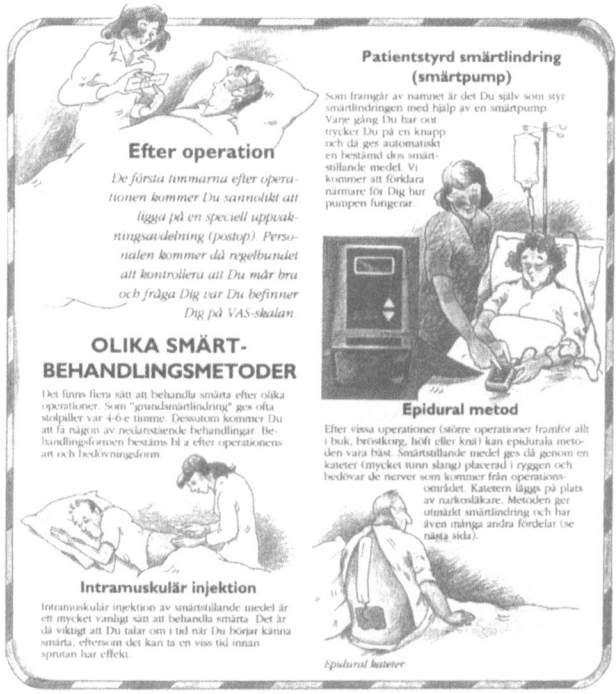

Fig. 2:
Pre-operative information provided to patients.

Floor discussion

In response to a comment by Rawal that more clinical studies are needed on the effects of dipyrone in post-operative pain, a number of participants offered comments on their experience with the drug. Professor H.G. Kress from Austria emphasized that he has used dipyrone for more than 20 years and has found it to be a very good alternative as the sole analgesic for children, as well as for severe pain in combination with opioids. This even holds true for the severe pain after thoracotomy in which dipyrone combined with tramadol is effective. A participant from Mexico agreed with Kress in that dipyrone is very useful in children, but also in chronic and cancer pain, for which 2 g dipyrone is given with diazepam. The side-effects of this combination are much less than those with morphine.

References

1. Warfield, C.A., Kahn, C.H., Acute pain management. Programs in U.S. hospitals and experiences and attitudes among US adults. Anesthesiology 83, 1090–1094 (1995).
2. Rawal, N., Regional analgesia and pain management in day surgery. European Society of Regional Anaesthesia meeting. Stockholm, August 25–27 1984. Barcelona, Permaneyer, 170–173 (1994).
3. Spence, A.A., Relieving acute pain (editorial), Br. J. Anaesth., 52, 245–246 (1980).
4. Mitchell, R.W.D. and Smith G., The control of acute postoperative pain, Br. J. Anaesth., 63, 147–158 (1989).
5. Oden, R.V., Acute postoperative pain: incidence, severity and the etiology of inadequate treatment, Anesth. Clin. N. Am. 7, 1–17 (1989).
6. International Association for the Study of Pain (IASP), Management of Acute Pain, A Practical Guide, Task Force on Acute Pain, L.B. Ready and W.T. Edwards, (Eds.), IASP Publications, 1992.
7. Rawal, N. and Berggren, L., Organization of acute pain services: a low-cost model. Pain 57, 117–123 (1994).
8. Monteus, M., A significant decrease of narcotic drug dosage after orthopedic surgery. A double-blind study with naproxen. Acta Orthopaed. Bel. 48, 900–902 (1982).
9. Pendeville, P.E., Van Boven, M.J., Contreras, V., et al., Ketorolac tromethamine for postoperative analgesia in oral surgery. Acta Anaesthesiol. Belg. 46, 25–30 (1995).
10. Dahl, J.B., Kehlet, H., Non-steroidal anti-inflammatory drugs: rationale for use in severe postoperative pain, Br. J. Anaesth. 66, 703–712 (1991).
11. Rusy, L.H., Houck, C.S., Sullivan, L.J., et al., A double-blind evaluation of ketolorac tromethamine versus acetaminophen in pediatric tonsillectomy: analgesia and bleeding, Anaesth. Analg. 80, 226–229 (1995).
12. Coderre, T.J., Katz, J., Vaccarino, A.L., Melzack, R., Contribution of central neuroplasticity to pathological pain: review of clinical and experimental evidence, Pain 52, 259–285 (1993).
13. Rawal, N., Analgesia technique and post-operative morbidity, Eur. I. Anaesth. 12 (Suppl. 10), 47–52 (1995).
14. Mourisse, J., Hasenbos, M.A.W.M., Gielen, M.J.M., et al., Epidural bupivacaine, sufentanil or the combination for post–thoracotomy pain. Acta Anaesthesiol. Scand. 36, 70–74 (1992).
15. George, K.A., Chisakuta, A.M., Gamble, J.A.S., Browne, G.A., Thoracic epidural infusion for postoperative pain relief following abdominal aortic surgery: bupivacaine, fentanyl or a mixture of both? Anaesthesia 47, 388–394 (1992).
16. Dahl, J.B., Rosenberg, J., Hansen, B.L. et al., Differential analgesic effects of low dose epidural morphine and morphine-bupivacaine at rest and during mobilization after major abdominal surgery. Anesth. Analg. 74, 362–365 (1992).
17. Hutchinson, G.L., Crofts, S.L., Gray, I.G., Preoperative piroxicam for postoperative analgesia in dental surgery, Br. J. Anaesth. 65, 500–503 (1990).

18. Manuksela, E.L., Olkkola, K., Korpela, R., Dose prophylactic intravenous infusion of indomethacin improve the management of postoperative pain in children? Can. J. Anaesth. *35*, 123–127 (1988).
19. Tigerstedt, I., Tammitso, T., Neuvonen, P.J., The efficacy of intravenous indomethacin in prevention of postoperative pain. Acta Anaesthesiol. Scand. *35*, 535–540 (1991).
20. Breivik, H., Pre-emptive analgesia. Curr. Opin. Anaesthesiol. *7*, 458–461 (1994).
21. Bridenbaugh, P.O., Pre-emptive analgesia – is it clinically relevant? Anesth. Analg. *78*, 203–204 (1994).

Non-opioid analgesics in cancer pain relief

Stephan A. Schug
Section of Anaesthetics,
Department of Pharmacology,
University of Auckland,
85 Park Road, Grafton,
Auckland, New Zealand

Introduction

Morphine and other strong opioids are the mainstay of cancer pain treatment. The development of new drug formulations and sophisticated delivery systems has further increased the flexibility of opioid therapy. What place, then, do non-opioids have in the management of cancer pain?

The step-ladder approach to the treatment of cancer pain, as advocated by the WHO, is now widely used (Fig. 1). As a first step, non-opioid

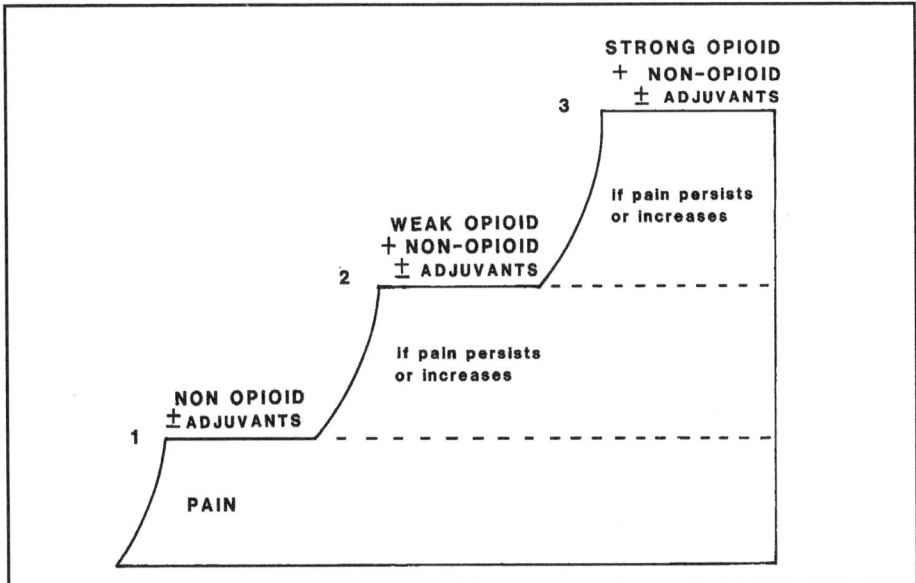

Fig. 1:
The WHO ladder approach to the treatment of cancer pain.

analgesics alone are recommended to treat mild to moderate pain. In case of persistent or increasing pain, a weak opioid is added to the regimen and the latter needs to be replaced, at the third step, with a strong opioid for severe pain. In view of the great variability in the intensity of cancer pain it is worth considering how many patients can be maintained at step one on the non-opioid analgesic alone. In a study performed in Cologne, we were able to show that at the time of admission to the pain clinic, non-opioids controlled pain in 20% of patients [1]. Subsequently, this proportion decreased to 5–7% of patients who could be maintained pain-free with non-opioid analgesics. As might be expected in the treatment of a progressive disease such as cancer, the use of opioids for severe pain increased continuously over time.

Nevertheless, even use of opioids requires co-administration of a non-opioid analgesic for maximum relief. Interestingly, in an analysis of 550 of our patients over 22,000 treatment days, the average daily oral morphine dose was only 82 mg, substantially lower than in other series reported in the literature [2]. Our conclusion was that the co-administration of non-opioids (mainly dipyrone and paracetamol), for 94% of the treatment time, was a major contributing factor to these relatively low opioid requirements. These findings suggest that non-opioids play a far larger role in cancer pain relief than is indicated by their sole use at step one of the WHO ladder.

Role of non-opioids in treatment of cancer pain

There are four main indications for non-opioid analgesics in the management of cancer pain. These are:
1. intercurrent pain, for example, in the cancer pain patient who is also suffering from migraine;
2. sole treatment for mild to moderate pain, as recommended at step one of the WHO ladder;
3. in combination with opioids at steps two and three of the WHO ladder;
4. for specific indications, such as the use of non-steroidal anti-inflammatory drugs (NSAIDs) for bone and soft-tissue pain or the use of dipyrone for visceral pain.

The non-opioids available for the relief of cancer pain are paracetamol, various NSAIDs and dipyrone. The benzoxazine analgesic, nefopam, has also been used for this purpose, but has no more efficacy than paracetamol, has marked anti-muscarinic side-effects and can cause sedation and confusion in a significant proportion of patients – particularly in the elderly [3]. We do not recommend, therefore, its use in this setting.

Paracetamol (acetaminophen)

Very few studies can be found in the literature regarding the use of this drug for cancer pain management. Presumably, because paracetamol is so widely available over-the-counter, it is considered neither interesting for the investigator nor economically viable for a pharmaceutical company to perform this sort of clinical study. Reference must be made, therefore, to the use of paracetamol in other types of pain.

In day-stay surgical patients randomised to take either 1 g paracetamol 4 hourly or 60 mg of a slow release preparation of dihydrocodeine 12 hourly, the number of patients who required rescue medication in the weak opioid group was twice as high as that in the paracetamol group (45% vs 22%) [4]. In addition, satisfaction scores were significantly higher in the paracetamol group. Despite the fact that this study involved postoperative rather than cancer pain patients, it serves to illustrate that paracetamol is an effective analgesic regardless of its widespread availability.

This impression is confirmed by a previous study on cancer pain published in 1981, which found aspirin and paracetamol to be equianalgesic and equipotent [5]. Little else can be concluded from the literature on paracetamol in cancer pain.

Despite the paucity of objective data, it is the practice of the Acute Pain Service at Auckland Hospital (and that of others – see chapter by N. Rawal) for all patients under our care (both acute and cancer pain patients) to receive background analgesia with 1 g paracetamol 4 hourly. We were able to confirm the value of this approach recently by a randomised blinded study in the postoperative setting. Patients using morphine via a PCA pump after orthopaedic surgery, who received additional paracetamol at the dosage given above, had lower pain scores, were able to discontinue morphine use earlier and were more satisfied with their analgesia than those on placebo [6].

The high bioavailability of paracetamol for oral administration makes it well suited for use in cancer pain. Documented side-effects of paracetamol are minor, it is well tolerated and has a high degree of patient acceptance.

Paracetamol taken in overdose is associated with irreversible liver damage. Recently, there has been growing concern about the potential for hepatotoxicity of paracetamol in therapeutic doses. This concern was primarily triggered by a publication on 67 cases of hepatic injury associated with paracetamol use [7]. All patients were heavy drinkers, 64 % of the patients were considered to be «alcoholic» or drinking more than 80 g of alcohol per day; thus this study describes a highly selected patient population. It is now recommended to be cautious with paracetamol usage in alcoholics and cachectic patients.

There are disadvantages in the use of paracetamol, however. Its analgesic efficacy is limited by a ceiling effect. The lack of a parenteral preparation of paracetamol in most countries (except France) also limits its indications.

Non-steroidal anti-inflammatory drugs (NSAIDs)

NSAIDs are well-established as sole analgesic agents for mild to moderate cancer pain or in combination with opioids for more severe pain .

An important question to raise is whether opioid-sparing *per se* provides any real advantage. Indeed, most clinical studies cannot demonstrate that opioid-sparing reduces the incidence of adverse events. Morphine is inexpensive, so the economic advantage of opioid-sparing with NSAIDs is negligible.

NSAIDs are considered to be of particular benefit in the treatment of pain associated with bone and soft tissue involvement. This is based on the fact that NSAIDs are inhibitors of prostaglandin synthesis and prostaglandins are not only mediators of inflammation but also of bone resorption [8]. However, while bone metastases are associated with pain, it has proved difficult to demonstrate a superior analgesic efficacy of NSAIDs in bone-related cancer pain, mainly because of the paucity of suitable studies [9].

Several studies have been performed in which the efficacy of NSAIDs in cancer pain has been investigated in a parallel, comparative manner. In a study by Stambaugh et al. [10], ibuprofen added to a combined preparation of oxycodone and paracetamol (available only in the United States) led to a further reduction in cancer pain intensity, improved pain relief scores and increased patient preference. Similarly, in another study, addition of 60 mg ibuprofen to either 2.5 or 5 mg methadone significantly increased the quality of analgesia [11], thereby demonstrating that the combination of a non-opioid and an opioid results not only in an opioid-sparing effect but also in improved analgesia.

In a recent meta-analysis of all available randomised, controlled trials on the use of NSAIDs in cancer pain, Eisenberg and colleagues [9] found that the analgesic efficacy of a single dose of an NSAID (indomethacin, ketoprofen or zomepirac) was equivalent to that of 5–10 mg intramuscular morphine. The meta-analysis revealed a dose-response relationship for NSAIDs in cancer pain up to a ceiling dose. This dose-response relationship also held true for side-effects. However, in this case, no ceiling effect was observed. Thus, the authors concluded that increasing the dose increased side-effects without enhancing analgesia. No single NSAID had any advantage over other members of this group of drugs. Interestingly, this meta-analysis provided no support for the WHO step two recommendation that the addition of an opioid for mild to moderate pain provides further improvement in analgesia above that provided by an NSAID.

NSAIDs have a specific side-effect profile closely related to their action as inhibitors of prostaglandin synthesis (Table 1); of particular importance are the adverse gastrointestinal and renal effects which present well-known risks in the clinical use of NSAIDs [12–14]. In the meta-analysis mentioned above [9], 34% of patients had upper gastrointestinal side-effects after a single NSAID dose, which increased to 44% on multiple dosing. The combination of NSAIDs with opioids for mild to moderate pain only increased the incidence of side-effects further.

Table 1:
Side effects of NSAIDs

- gastric ulceration
- impairment of platelet function
- impairment of renal function
- impairment of healing
- induction of bronchospasm

It can be concluded that NSAIDs have a proven analgesic effect and are probably more potent than paracetamol, although definitive data are currently lacking. Theoretically, NSAIDs offer an additional anti-inflammatory effect as well as their analgesic action in cancer pain. However, it is not clear how this contributes towards efficacy in practice. The specific adverse effects of NSAIDs provide a significant limitation to their use as analgesics. As a result, there is a clear need for a potent, non-opioid analgesic with minimal gastrointestinal side-effects. Dipyrone would appear to fill this therapeutic gap.

Dipyrone

In postoperative pain, dipyrone is more effective as an analgesic than paracetamol [15] (Fig. 2). The analgesic response to 1 g dipyrone given intramuscularly is equivalent to that of 100 mg pethidine or 10 mg morphine [16]. The additional intrinsic spasmolytic action of dipyrone may also be of value in the treatment of specific types of cancer pain in which muscle spasm is involved, such as visceral pain [17].

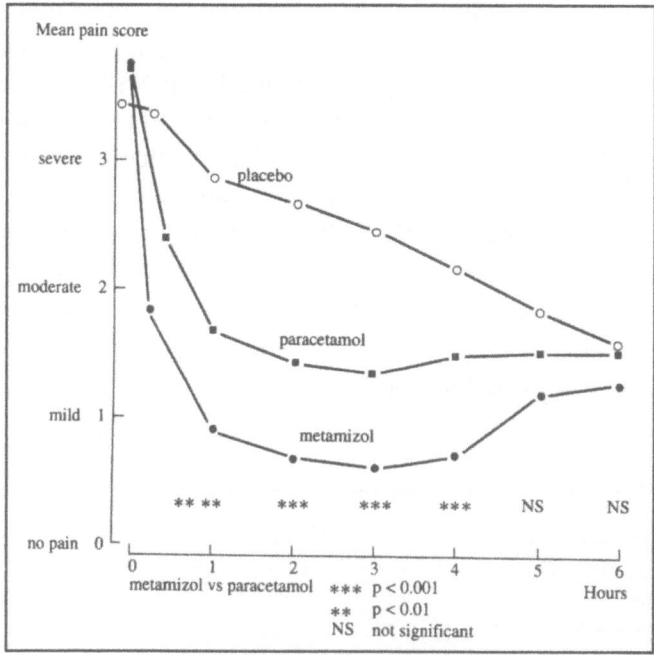

Fig. 2: Comparison of the effect of placebo, paracetamol and dipyrone on postoperative pain (modified from [20]).

Only one study has been reported on the use of dipyrone in chronic cancer pain [18]. Patients were given 6 g oral dipyrone daily in three divided doses. Over a 7 day treatment period, the pain relief achieved was comparable to that obtained with 10 mg oral morphine given every 4 hours. These data indicate that in a cancer pain population which requires treatment with up to 60 mg oral morphine per day, the same analgesic effect can be achieved with the non-opioid, dipyrone.

On the basis of current knowledge, dipyrone may be seen as a potent alternative to paracetamol and can be used as the sole analgesic in some cancer pain patients or in combination with opioids. It may also be regarded as a suitable specific co-analgesic in patients with spasm or visceral pain.

Dipyrone has negligible effects on peripheral prostaglandin synthesis and therefore is not associated with the NSAID-specific gastrointestinal and renal side-effects. A further advantage of dipyrone is its availability in oral (tablets and suspension), intravenous and rectal preparations.

Table 2:
Dipyrone in the management of cancer pain

Advantages:
–   more potent than paracetamol
–   proven spasmolytic effect
–   oral, rectal, parenteral preparations available
–   no NSAID-specific side-effects

Limitations:
–   no relevant anti-inflammatory effect
–   clinical trial data still insufficient
–   not universally available

Conclusions

The role of non-opioid analgesics in the management of cancer pain is widely underestimated. They are the sole analgesics for intercurrent pain and in step one of the WHO analgesic ladder for the treatment of mild to moderate cancer pain. In addition, non-opioid analgesics can reduce both opioid requirements and side-effects and may improve analgesia in severe cancer pain at steps 2 and 3 of the WHO analgesic ladder. Some non-opioid analgesics may have specific indications in the treatment of cancer pain: NSAIDs for inflammatory bone and soft tissue pain and dipyrone for visceral pain (spasms).

Currently available non-opioid analgesics have therapeutic limitations in the management of cancer pain because of their analgesic ceiling effect, their side-effect profiles and the restricted routes of administration which can be used. Dipyrone may fill some of these gaps in our current therapeutic armamentarium.

Floor discussion

A physician commented that he had a patient who came to his clinic who was controlling his pain on 30 g dipyrone daily without side-effects. Dr. Schug emphasized that this dose was far too high but he agreed that paracetamol and dipyrone are well-tolerated analgesics. He regularly uses 6 g paracetamol in the treatment of post-operative pain.

Asked if he would recommend the use of 6 g dipyrone for visceral pain, Dr. Schug replied that use of 60 mg oral morphine is approximately equivalent to use of 6 g oral dipyrone daily. In referring to the cancer pain study in which this dose of dipyrone was used, he emphasized that dipyrone has a ceiling effect, but the ceiling for cancer pain management is not yet clear.

In response to a comment about the small amount of data on the use of dipyrone in cancer pain, Dr. Schug pointed out that studies on paracetamol and cancer pain do not even exist.

References

1. Schug, S.A., Zech, D., Doerr, U., Cancer pain management according to WHO Analgesic Guidelines in the course of time. J. Pain Symptom Manage. 5, 27-32 (1990).
2. Schug, S.A., Zech, D., Grond, S., et al., A long-term survey of morphine in cancer pain patients. J. Pain Symptom Manage. 7, 259–266 (1992).
3. Drage, M.P., Schug, S.A., Analgesia in the elderly – Practical treatment recommendations. Drugs Aging 9, 311–318 (1996).
4. Schug, S.A., Payne, J.P., Dijkhuizen, M.R.J., Routine analgesia after day stay surgery: slow release dihydrocodeine compared with paracetamol. Abstracts 8th World Congress of Pain, IASP Press, Seattle 267 (1996).
5. Cooper, S.A., Comparative analgesic efficacies of aspirin and acetaminophen. Arch. Intern. Med. 141, 282–285 (1981).

6. Sidebotham, D.A., Schug, S.A., McGuinnety, M., Fox, L., The addition of acetaminophen to patient controlled analgesia in the management of acute postoperative pain. Abstract submitted for presentation at 22nd Annual Meeting of ASRA, Atlanta (1997).

7. Zimmerman, H.J., Maddrey, W.C., Acetaminophen hepatotoxicity with regular intake of alcohol: analysis of instances of therapeutic misadventure. Hepatology 22, 767–773 (1995).

8. Seyberth, H.W., Prostaglandin-mediated hypercalcemia: a paraneoplastic syndrome. Klin. Wschr. 56, 373–387 (1978).

9. Eisenberg, E., Berkey, C.S., Carr, D.B., Mosteller, F., Chalmers, T.C., Efficacy and safety of nonsteroidal antiinflammatory drugs for cancer pain: a meta-analysis. J. Clin. Oncol. 12, 2756–2765 (1994).

10. Stambaugh, J.E., Drew, J., The combination of ibuprofen and oxycodone/ acetaminophen in the treatment of chronic cancer pain. Clin. Pharmacol. Ther. 44, 665–669 (1988).

11. Ferrer-Brechner, T., Ganz, P., Combination therapy with ibuprofen and methadone for chronic cancer pain. Am. J. Med. 77, 78–83 (1984).

12. Kaufman, D.W., Kelly, J.P., Sheehan, J.E., et al., Nonsteroidal anti-inflammatory drug use in relation to major upper gastrointestinal bleeding. Clin. Pharmacol. Ther. 53, 485–494 (1993).

13. García Rodríguez, L.A., Jick, H., Risk of upper gastrointestinal bleeding and perforation associated with individual non-steroidal anti-inflammatory drugs. Lancet 343, 769–772 (1994).

14. Langman, M.J.S., Weil, J., Wainwright, P., et al., Risks of bleeding peptic ulcer associated with individual non-steroidal anti-inflammatory drugs. Lancet 343, 1075–1078 (1994).

15. Gomez-Jiminez, J., Franco-Patino, R., Chargoy-Vera, J., Olivares-Sosa, R., Clinical efficacy of mild analgesics in pain following gynaecological or dental surgery. Br. J. Clin. Pharmac. 10, 355S–358S (1980).

16. Patel, C.V., Koppikar, M.G., Patel, M.S., Parulkar, G.B., Pinto-Pereira, L.M., Management of pain after abdominal surgery: dipyrone compared with pethidine. Br. J. Clin. Pharmacol. 10, 351S–354S (1980).

17. Miralles, R., Cami, J., Gutierrez, J., et al, Diclofenac versus dipyrone in acute renal colic; a double-blind controlled trial. Eur. J. Clin. Pharm. 33, 527–528 (1987).

18. Rodríguez, M., Barutell, C., Rull, M., et al., Efficacy and tolerance of oral dipyrone versus oral morphine for cancer pain. Eur. J. Cancer 30A, 584–587 (1994).

Comparative safety of non-opioid analgesics

Carlos Martinez,
Hoechst Marion Roussel
Hoechst AG
D-65926 Frankfurt a.M., Germany

The purpose of the evaluation described in this chapter was to estimate and to compare the adverse drug-attributed, public health impact of dipyrone with that of other non-narcotic analgesics (NNAs) and non-steroidal anti-inflammatory drugs (NSAIDs) which have similar indications and duration of use. Such a comparative safety evaluation must employ an objective measure in order to incorporate, quantify and weigh the impact of all adverse events (AEs). A suitable common outcome measure, however, will depend on the perspective chosen. Ideally, such an evaluation should take into account all known drug-attributed AEs, their duration and frequency of occurrence and their varying degrees of severity.

The following evaluation was made from an epidemiologic perspective. The possibility of death was chosen as the common outcome of the different AEs, thereby restricting the evaluation to potentially life-threatening AEs. As a result, it has been possible to estimate the drug-related mortality expected from the short-term administration of dipyrone, other NNAs and NSAIDs. The adverse drug-attributed public health impact of each drug was expressed as the overall excess mortality or the expected number of deaths due to all adverse events per million cases per week.

Methods

All potentially fatal AEs reported with NNAs and NSAIDs were identified as anaphylaxis, Stevens-Johnson syndrome and toxic epidermal necrolysis (SJS/TEN), agranulocytosis, aplastic anemia, upper gastrointestinal complications (hemorrhage and/or perforations) (see Fig. 1). A search of the English language literature was performed using the Medline database to locate all epidemiologic studies published from January, 1970 to December, 1995 in which association of these potentially fatal AEs with the use of NNAs (including paracetamol and dipyrone) and NSAIDs was investigated.

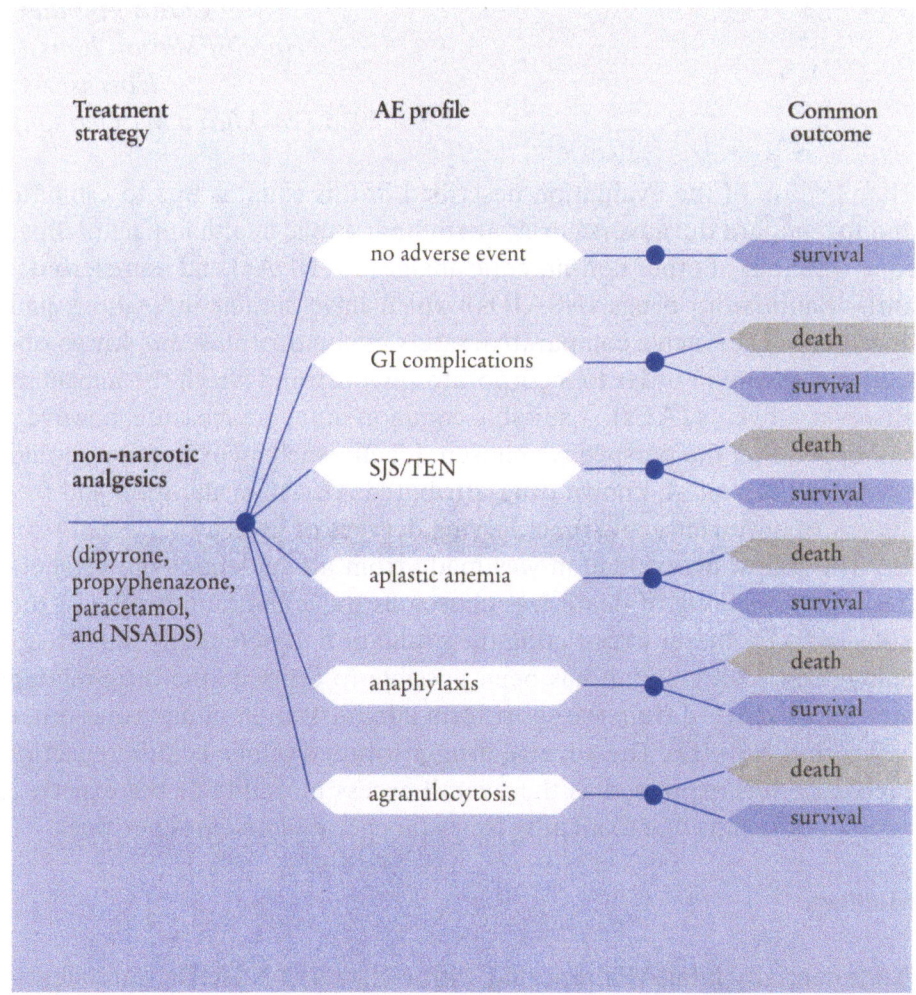

Fig. 1:
Potentially fatal adverse events (AEs) to non-narcotic analgesics and their common outcome.

All case-control or cohort studies were selected which permitted a calculation of the excess mortality in the population studied. For case-control studies, the required data included estimates of the relative risk associated with drug exposure compared to non-exposure, the percentage of cases exposed to the drug, the overall incidence rate of the relevant diseases in the source population, and the respective case-fatality rate (proportion of subjects with the AE who died). When necessary data were not included in the original article, a Medline literature search was performed to locate auxiliary reports by the study investigators which presented estimates of the overall risk of the relevant diseases in terms of estimates of the case-fatality rate. For each study, the AE-specific excess mortality attributed to short-term administration (a one week period) of a defined drug was calculated by multiplying the estimate of the one-week excess risk by the respective case-fatality rate. One week risks of disease in the general population were determined from risk estimates for longer time periods under the assumption of a constant risk of disease.

The excess mortality was summed across AEs to determine the overall excess mortality attributed to short-term use of each NNA and NSAID. When more than one study was located in which the association between an agent and a given AE was assessed, the median excess mortality estimate for the agent was used.

Results

Eleven case-control studies contained the necessary information to calculate five AE-specific excess mortality rates attributed to NNAs and NSAIDs: one study on anaphylaxis [1], one on SJS/TEN [2], one on agranulocytosis [3], one on aplastic anemia [3], and seven studies on serious gastrointestinal complications including hemorrhage and perforations [4–10]. The different NNAs and NSAIDs investigated in the 11 studies are given in Table 1.

Only for dipyrone, paracetamol, aspirin and diclofenac was the necessary information available for all five AEs identified. Nevertheless, excess mortality rates were calculated for all NNAs (dipyrone, propyphenazone and paracetamol) and for NSAIDs (aspirin, diclofenac, indomethacin, naproxen, ibuprofen, piroxicam, ketoprofen, azapropazone, fenbufen and diflunisal), which were investigated in at least one gastrointestinal complication study.

Table 1:
Excess mortality per million in users of NNAs and NSAIDs

	Agranulocytosis	Aplastic Anemia	Anaphylaxis	SJS/TEN	GI bleeding	Total
NNAs						
Dipyrone	0.039	0.000	0.002	0.002	0.171	**0.21**
Paracetamol	0.0013	0.006	0.0007	0.023	0.190	**0.22**
Propyphenazone	0.0013	0.000	0.0007		0.000	**0.002**
NSAIDs						
Aspirin	0.006	0.003	0.002	0.002	1.839	**1.9**
Diflunisal					10.183	**10.2**
Azapropazone					57.539	**57.5**
Diclofenac	0.000	0.054	0.004	0.011	5.857	**5.9**
Fenbufen					1.195	**1.2**
Ibuprofen				0.004	5.308	**5.3**
Indomethacin	0.035	0.120			11.576	**11.7**
Ketoprofen				0.004	23.286	**23.3**
Naproxen			0.002	0.004	6.474	**6.5**
Piroxicam		0.109		0.064	21.066	**21.2**

Of the seven studies in which serious gastrointestinal complications were examined, three studies [5,8,10] restricted the analyses to hospitalizations and/or deaths due to bleeding or perforated peptic ulcer, and another study [9] provided data on bleeding exclusively due to peptic ulcer. For five studies [5–9] the estimates of the overall incidence and/or the case-fatality of the gastrointestinal complications were obtained from auxiliary reports [11–15]. Incidence data and case-fatality rates for SJS/TEN were identified from auxiliary reports as well [16,17].

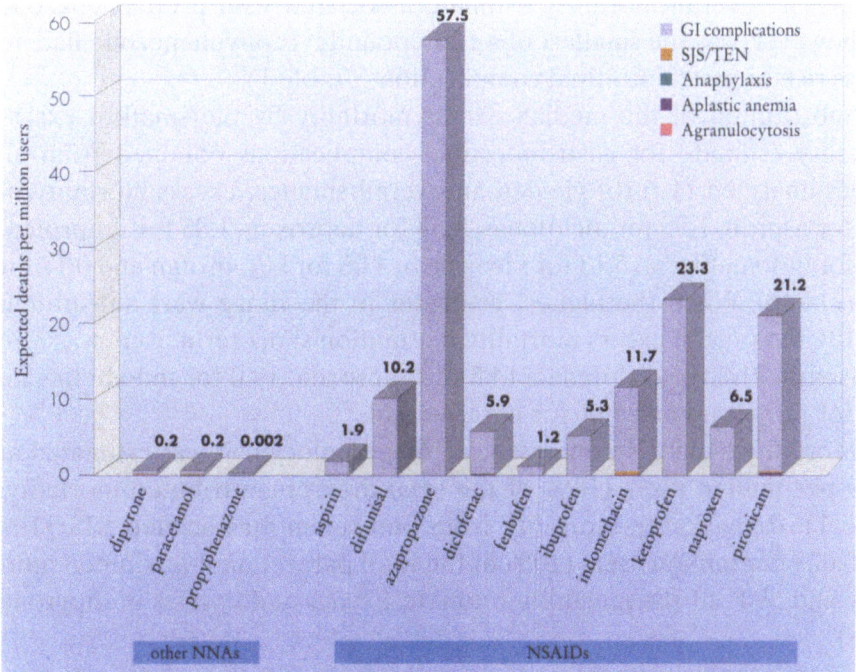

Fig. 2:
Overall mortality attributed to NNAs and NSAIDs.

The overall excess mortality from anaphylaxis, SJS/TEN, agranulocytosis, aplastic anemia, and serious upper gastrointestinal complications was higher for NSAIDs than for NNAs (Table1, Fig. 2). Using the mean excess mortality estimates, for NSAIDs the mortality per million users over a one-week period was 1.20 for fenbufen, 1.85 for aspirin, 5.31 for ibuprofen,

5.93 for diclofenac, 6.48 for naproxen, 11.7 for indomethacin, 21.2 for piroxicam, 23.3 for ketoprofen and 57.5 for azapropazone. Among NNAs, the mortality per million users over a one week period ranged from 0.002 for propyphenazone to 0.214 for dipyrone and 0.221 for paracetamol users, respectively (Table 1, Fig. 2). The excess mortality associated with gastrointestinal complications was the major determinant of the overall estimate, contributing to 99% of the excess mortality in users of all NSAIDs. The major determinant of the overall estimate in users of NNAs was gastrointestinal complications for paracetamol users (86%) and dipyrone users (80%). The overall mortality estimate associated with propyphenazone use, however, was the smallest of all compounds. Propyphenazone had no excess risk of gastrointestinal complications (Table 1).

Substitution of the median excess mortality by the smallest excess mortality estimate for gastrointestinal complications obtained from all studies analyzed [4–6,10] yielded an overall smallest excess mortality of 0.75 for aspirin, 1.95 for diclofenac, 1.57 for naproxen, 1.85 for ibuprofen, 1.26 for indomethacin, 5.13 for piroxicam, 4.08 for ketoprofen and 0.17 for paracetamol. When the highest estimates in the range were substituted [5,7,10], the overall excess mortality per million short-term users was 3.26 for aspirin, 21.2 for diclofenac, 14.5 for naproxen, 19.0 for indomethacin, 23.4 for piroxicam and 0.66 for paracetamol.

Mortality from dipyrone-associated agranulocytosis was estimated at 0.039 per million users (18% of the total dipyrone-attributed mortality; Table 1). Remarkably, mortality from paracetamol-associated SJS/TEN was 0.023 per million users (10% of the total paracetamol-attributed mortality and 59% of the mortality estimate for agranulocytosis in dipyrone users).

To test the robustness of the results, a sensitivity analysis was performed in which estimated mortality was evaluated for different estimates of the overall annual incidence rate of agranulocytosis. The overall annual incidence rate of agranulocytosis from studies published after 1970 ranged from 1.5 in Milan (1980–1986) to 29.8 in the Stockholm county region (1973–1975). Table 2 summarizes the annual incidence rates of agranulocytosis from different sources [3,20–23]. The inclusion of the highest annual estimate of 29.8 per million would result in an overall excess mortality estimate for dipyrone of 0.83, which is still much smaller than for any other

Table 2:
Community-acquired agranulocytosis

Investigator	Dates	Method, Study design	Country	Size	Cases (N)	IR per million
Kaufman [3]	1980-1986	Population-based case-control study	**Europe, Israel (total)**	22.3	380	3.4
			Ulm, Germany	5.2	63	2.9
			Berlin, Germany	1.8	28	2.0
			Barcelona	4.1	78	3.2
			Israel	3.9	72	3.7
			Budapest	2.0	64	5.5
			Stockholm/Uppsala	1.8	45	5.1
			Milan	2.3	13	1.5
			Sofia	1.1	17	3.8
Strom [20]	1980-1983	Medicaid billing data overall 7.2 per million	**Three states (total)**		20	7.2
	1980-1983		Minnesota		2	2.3
	1980-1983		Michigan		16	7.7
	1983		Florida		2	15.4
Arneborn* [21]	1973-1975	Hospital discharge diagnosis	Stockholm county region	1.49	133	29.8
Kantero* [22]	1966-1967	Hospital discharge diagnosis (children under 15)	Helsinki	1.2	13	5.4
Palva [23]	1967-1968	Hospital discharge diagnosis (children under 15)	Helsinki, Oulu	0.4	4	10.0

* agranulocytosis defined as granulocyte count of less than 1000/mm [3]
IR = incidence rate

NSAID. Furthermore, the overall annual incidence rate of agranulocytosis would need to exceed 75 and 264 per million, i.e. 22 and 78 times the incidence rate as estimated in the IAAAS [3], for the overall excess mortality of dipyrone to be comparable to the overall excess mortality associated with aspirin and diclofenac, respectively. By analogy, the relative risk estimate for the association of dipyrone with agranulocytosis would have to exceed an excess mortality of 310 to be comparable to that of aspirin and 1200 to be comparable to that of diclofenac.

Assuming similar benefits of all non-narcotic analgesics and defining the diclofenac-associated mortality as baseline, Fig. 3 provides the incremental number of deaths per million drug users.

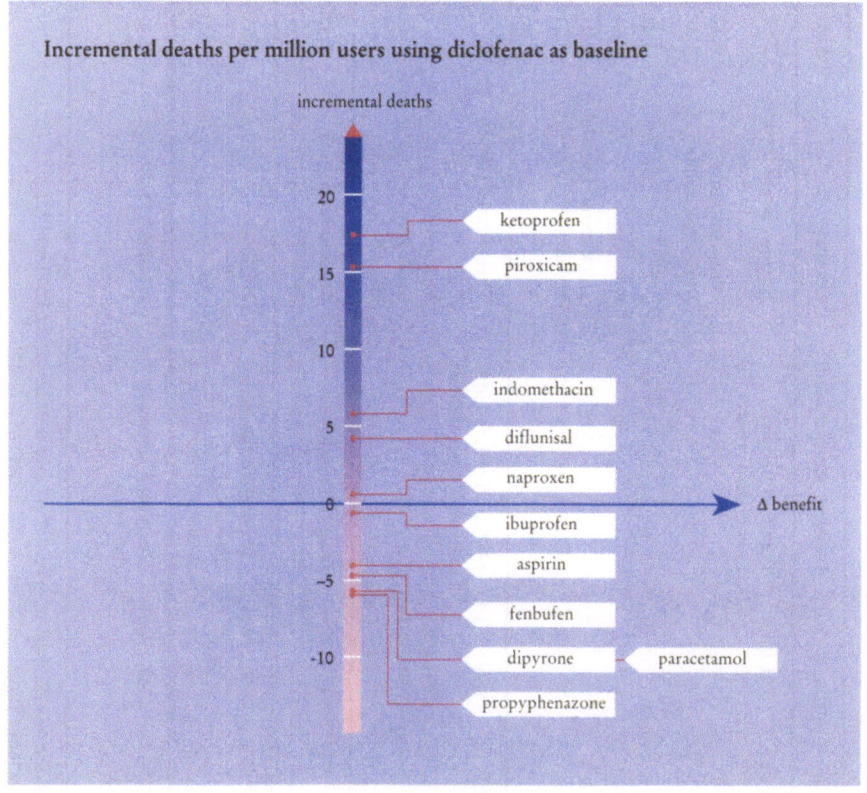

Fig. 3:
Incremental deaths per million users using diclofenac as baseline.

Discussion

The results of this evaluation show that overall excess mortality estimates are largely influenced by the excess mortality associated with upper gastrointestinal complications, an AE more commonly associated with the use of NSAIDs, such as aspirin, diclofenac or naproxen, than with the use of dipyrone or any other NNA. Agranulocytosis, aplastic anemia, anaphylaxis and SJS/TEN proved to be extremely uncommon conditions and to have practically no public health impact in terms of drug-related mortality.

Estimates of the overall annual incidence of a number of additional AEs reported in association with the use of one or more of the analgesics evaluated [6,16,24–34]. The estimated baseline mortality rates associated with each of these diseases (including acute pancreatitis, acute liver injury and acute toxin-induced renal failure), which have rarely been reported on short-term use of the analgesics evaluated, are 10 to 20–fold less than that associated with severe upper gastrointestinal complications. Thus, it is unlikely that further evaluation of these events would have any impact on the overall study results.

Several limitations are apparent in the evaluation of total risk associated with drug therapies. The restriction of the analysis to studies with a case-control or a cohort study design which provided data suitable for assessing the excess mortality in the population studied may have influenced the findings. Considerable heterogeneity in the estimates of excess mortality due to upper gastrointestinal complications existed between studies, resulting from the disparate estimates of relative risk, total incidence in the population, and the percent of patients exposed to the agent under evaluation. The data necessary for the evaluation of the precision of the overall risk estimates were not available for many of the studies, precluding appropriate assessment of the precision of the excess mortality estimates and the differences between the estimates. For diclofenac, the relative risk estimates for the association with upper gastrointestinal complications included in the analyses were somewhat higher than those generally observed in epidemiologic investigations [35–43]. These relative risk estimates, however, were associated with smaller case-fatality rates and with a smaller excess mortality rate.

Another limitation of the present evaluation was the use of relative risk estimates that did not account for the duration of therapy, drug dose, or previous therapy with the drugs under investigation. In this case, it was assumed that the risk of adverse effects was constant throughout therapy, which is unlikely. For anaphylaxis, the majority of reactions occurs within one hour after drug exposure [18–19]. Variability in the risk of agranulocytosis and aplastic anemia over a course of drug therapy is also likely.

The risk of gastrointestinal hemorrhage is highest early during nonsteroidal anti-inflammatory drug therapy (within 1 month after initiation) and decreases with time [45,46]. Patients who started taking aspirin one week before hospital admission for GI bleeding had an increased relative risk of 4.8 when compared to the constant relative risk of 2.9 associated with prior aspirin intake of between one week and three months. This observation receives further support from a process termed «gastric mucosal adaptation». Despite continuous administration of injurious compounds (e.g. aspirin) over several days, gastric mucosal damage is seen to decrease. Chronic injury is associated with a more accelerated mucosal healing process than is acute injury. In humans, gastric adaptation has been shown to occur in response to aspirin and indomethacin administration. Visible gastric mucosal damage reached a maximum within one and three days of indomethacin and aspirin administration, respectively. Mucosal damage tended to resolve despite continued intake of the injurious compounds [46–49].

Experimental studies in humans have also shown a clear dose-response relationship in the time required for the resolution of mucosal injury. The time required was longer at a higher dose of aspirin [46]. Prophylactic use of 75 mg aspirin per day has been shown to increase significantly the risk of peptic ulcer bleeding [44].

In the present study, adverse drug-attributed public health impact was estimated by using death as the common outcome of the different AEs. A more comprehensive risk evaluation, however, would need to consider the consequences of non-fatal AEs. Once a common outcome measure for non-fatal AEs has been developed, the approach presented here could be expanded.

Conclusions

In order to compare the adverse drug-attributed public health impact of short-term use of non-narcotic analgesics (NNAs) and non-steroidal anti-inflammatory drugs (NSAIDs) an epidemiologic perspective was chosen and the drug-related mortality quantified.

The expected mortality associated with dipyrone use appears to be comparable to that expected with paracetamol use and substantially lower than the risk associated with NSAID use for short term pain relief. The estimated excess mortality due to five potentially fatal AEs, i.e. agranulocytosis, aplastic anemia, anaphylaxis, SJS/TEN and serious upper gastrointestinal complications, was 1.20 for fenbufen, 1.85 for aspirin, 5.31 for ibuprofen, 5.93 for diclofenac, 6.48 for naproxen, 11.7 for indomethacin, 21.2 for piroxicam, 23.2 for ketoprofen and 57.5 for azapropazone per million users. Among NNAs, the mortality per million users ranged from 0.002 for propyphenazone to 0.214 for dipyrone and 0.221 for paracetamol users, respectively.

The excess mortality associated with gastrointestinal complications made the major contribution to the overall estimate, accounting for 99% or more of the excess mortality in NSAID users. In NNA users, such as dipyrone and paracetamol, the adverse event contributing the most to the overall mortality estimate was gastrointestinal complications as well, accounting for 80% and 86% of overall mortality, respectively. NNA-related mortality due to gastrointestinal-bleeding, however, is at least ten-fold less than NSAID-related mortality to the same cause.

It can be concluded that the public health impact of adverse effects of NNAs, including dipyrone, is at least ten-fold lower than for NSAIDs. Thus, when the choice of treatment is either an NNA or an NSAID, the use of an NNA such as dipyrone or paracetamol is to be recommended.

Floor discussion

Dr. Martinez was asked how other companies have responded to the data he has obtained. In his reply, Dr. Martinez emphasized the novelty of the approach taken in his investigation which permits, for the first time, a comparison of totally distinct adverse events. Dr. Martinez commented that

other colleagues have asked whether the approach can be used for drugs other than analgesics. Provided that studies can be obtained from the literature which fulfill the predetermined criteria, the approach should be applicable to any class of drugs.

Responding to the request of a participant from Egypt for retrospective studies of risks with analgesics in cancer patients, Martinez did not think that the risks would change when looking retrospectively. The large number of patients covered by his data made the risk calculations quite accurate. Because of the overwhelming predominance of gastrointestinal complications with non-opioid analgesics, it is unlikely that retrospective studies would significantly change the low incidence of other side-effects such as agranulocytosis.

Asked what would happen if the calculations were made for a 1-3 month treatment duration, instead of 1 week treatment, Martinez replied that few studies are available on long-term treatment. Moreover, agranulocytosis and anaphylaxis either occur early or not at all. As far as gastrointestinal bleeding is concerned, the risk remains high on chronic treatment with analgesics, but decreases after 2–3 weeks treatment. Consequently, calculation of risks of adverse events with analgesic use for a longer period would not provide additional relevant data to those obtained using a 1 week treatment period.

References

1. van der Klauw, M.M., Stricker, B.H.C., Herings, RMC, Cost, W.S., Valkenburg, H.A., Wilson, H.P., A population based case-cohort study of drug-induced anaphylaxis. Br. J. Clin. Pharmac. *35*, 400–408 (1993).
2. Roujeau, J.C., Kelly, J.P., Naldi, L., et al., Drug etiology of Stevens-Johnson syndrome and toxic epidemal necrolysis, first results from an international case-control study. N. Engl. J. Med. *333*, 1600–1609 (1995).
3. Kaufman, D.W., Kelly, J.P., Levy, M., Shapiro, S., The drug etiology of agranulo-cytosis and aplastic anemia. Monographs in Epidemiology and Biostatistics. Volume 18, Oxford University Press 1991.
4. Laporte, J.R., Carné, X., Vidal, X., Moreno, V., Juan, J., Upper gastrointestinal bleeding in relation to previous use of analgesics and non-steroidal anti-inflammatory drugs. Lancet *337*, 85–89 (1991).
5. Langman, M.J.S., Weil, J., Wainwright, P., et al., Risks of bleeding peptic ulcer associated with individual non-steroid anti-inflammatory drugs. Lancet *343*, 1075–1078 (1994).

6. Henry, D., Dobson, A., Turner, C., Variability in the risk of major gastrointestinal complications from nonaspirin nonsteroidal anti-inflammatory drugs. Gastroenterol. *105*, 1078–1088 (1993).

7. Langman, M.J.S., Coggon, D., Spiegelhalter, D., Analgesic intake and the risk of acute upper gastrointestinal bleeding. Am. J. Med. *74*, 79–82 (1983).

8. Faulkner, G., Prichard, P., Somerville, K., Langman, M.J.S., Aspirin and bleeding peptic ulcers in the elderly. Br. Med. J. *297*, 1311–1313 (1988).

9. Needham, C.D., Kyle, J., Jones, P.F., Johnston, S.J., Kerridge, D.F., Aspirin and alcohol in gastrointestinal haemorrhage. Gut, *12*, 819–821 (1971).

10. Armstrong, C.P., Blower, A.L., Non-steroidal anti-inflammatory drugs and life threatening complications of peptic ulceration. Gut *28*, 527–532 (1987).

11. Johnston, S.J., Jones, P.F., Kyle, J., Needham, C.D., Epidemiology and course of gastrointestinal haemorrhage in north-east Scotland. Br. Med. J. *3*, 655–660 (1973).

12. Somerville, K., Faulkner, G., Langman, M., Non-steroidal anti-inflammatory drugs and bleeding peptic ulcer. Lancet *i*, 462–464 (1986).

13. Katschinski, B.D., Logan, R.F.A., Davies, J., Langman, M.J.S., Audit of mortality in upper gastrointestinal bleeding. Postgrad. Med. J. *65*, 913–917 (1989).

14. Henry, D., Robertson, J., Nonsteroidal anti-inflammatory drugs and peptic ulcer hospitalization rates in New South Wales. Gastroenterol. *104*, 1083–1091 (1993).

15. Henry, D.A., Johnston, A., Dobson, A., Duggan, J., Fatal peptic ulcer complications and the use of non-steroidal anti-inflammatory drugs, aspirin, and corticosteroids. Br. Med. J. *295*, 1227–1229 (1987).

16. Schöpf, E., Rzany, B., Mockenhaupt M: Schwere arzneimittelinduzierte Hautreaktionen: Pemphigus vulgaris, bullöses Pemphigoid, generalized bullous fixed drug eruption, Erythema exsudativum multiforme majus, Stevens-Johnson-Syndrom und toxischepidermale Nekrolyse. Fortschr. prakt. Dermatol. Venerol. 89–95 (1994).

17. Mockenhaupt, M., Schligmann, J., Schröder, W., Schöpf, E., Evaluation of non-steroidal anti-inflammatory drugs (NSAIDs) and muscle relaxants as risk factors for Stevens-Johnson Syndrom (SJS) and toxic epidermal necrolysis (TEN). Pharmacoepidemiol. Drug Safety *5*, S116 (1996).

18. Bochner, B.S., Lichtenstein, L.M., Anaphylaxis. N. Engl. J. Med. *324*, 1785–1790 (1991).

19. Wasserman, S.I., Marquardt, D.L., Anaphylaxis. In: Middleton, E. Jr., Reed, C.E., Ellis, E.F., Adkinson, N.F.Jr., Yunginger, J.W. (eds.) Allergy: principles and practice. Vol.2. St. Louis, C.V. Mosby, 1365–79 (1988).

20. Strom, B.L., Carson, J.L., Schinnar, R., Snyder, E.S., Shaw, M., Descriptive epidemiology of agranulocytosis. Arch. Intern. Med. *152*, 1475–1480 (1992).

21. Arneborn, P., Palmblad, J., Drug-induced neutropenia: A survey for Stockholm 1973–1978. Acta Med. Scand. *212*, 289–292 (1982).

22. Kantero, I., Mustala, O.O., Drug-induced agranulocytosis, with special reference to aminophenazone. Acta Med. Scand. *192*, 327–330 (1972).

23. Palva, I.P., Mustala, O.O., Palva, I.P., Drug-induced agranulocytosis, with special reference to aminophenazone. I. Adults. Acta Med. Scand. *187*, 109–115 (1970).

24. Thomson, S.R., Hendry, W.S., McFarlane, G.A., Davidson, A.I., Epidemiology and outcome of acute pancreatitis. Br. J. Surg. *74*, 398–401 (1987).

25. Mann, D.V., Hershman, M.J., Hittinger, R., Glazer, G., Multicentre audit of death from acute pancreatitis. Br. J. Surg. *81*, 890–893 (1994).

26. Carson, J.L., Strom, B.L., Duff, A., Gupta, A., Dasm, K., Safety of nonsteroidal anti-inflammatory drugs with respect to acute liver disease. Arch. Int. Med. *153*, 1331–1336 (1993).

27. Garcia Rodriguez, L.A., Pérez Gutthann, S., Walker, A.M., Lueck, L., The role of non-steroidal anti-inflammatory drugs in acute liver injury. Br. Med. J, *305*, 865–868 (1992).
28. Mary, J.Y., Baumelou, E., Guiguet, M., Epidemiology of aplastic anemia in France: A prospective multicentric study. Blood 75, 1646–1653 (1990).
29. Nuyts, G.D., Elseviers, M.M., De Broe, M.E., Health impact of renal disease due to nephrotoxicity. Toxicol. Letters *46*, 31–44 (1989).
30. Lauwerys, R., Bernard, A., Preclinical detection of nephrotoxicity: description of the tests and appraisal of their health significance. Toxicol. Letters *46*, 13–29 (1989).
31. McMurray, S.D., Luft, F.C., Maxwell, D.R., et al., Prevailing patterns and predictor variables in patients with acute tubular necrosis. Arch. Intern. Med. *138*, 950–955 (1978).
32. Roujeau, J.C., Guillaume, J.C., Fabre, J.P., Penso, D., Flechet, M.L., Girre, J.P., Toxic epidermal necrolysis (Lyell Syndrome). Incidence and drug etiology in France, 1981–1985. Arch. Dermatol. *126*, 37–42 (1990).
33. Chan, H.L., Stern, R.S., Arndt, K.A., et al., The incidence of erythema multiforme, Stevens-Johnson Syndrome, and toxic epidermal necrolysis. Arch. Dermatol. *126*, 43–47 (1990).
34 Strom, B.L., Carson, J.L., Halpern, A.C., et al., A population-based study of Stevens-Johnson Syndrome. Arch. Dermatol. *127*, 831–838 (1991).
35. Savage, R.L., Moller, P.W., Ballantyne, C.L., Wells, J.E., Variation in the risk of peptic ulcer complications with nonsteroidal antiinflammatory drug therapy. Arth. Rheum. *36*, 84–90 (1993).
36. Kaufman, D.W., Kelly, J.P., Sheehan, J.E., et al., Nonsteroidal anti-inflammatory drug use in relation to major upper gastrointestinal bleeding. Clin. Pharmacol. Ther. *53*, 485–494 (1993).
37. Garcia Rodriguez, L.A., Walker, A.M., Pérez Gutthann, S., Nonsteroidal antiinflammatory drugs and gastrointestinal hospitalizations in Sasketchewan: A cohort study. Epidemiol. *3*, 337–342 (1992).
38. Nobili, A., Mosconi, P., Franzosi, M.G., Tognoni, G., Non-steroidal anti-inflammatory drugs and upper gastrointestinal bleeding, a post-marketing surveillance case-control study. Pharmacoepidemiol. Drug Safety *1*, 65–72 (1992).
39. Garcia Rodriguez, L.A., Jick, H., Risk of upper gastrointestinal bleeding and perforation associated with individual non-steroidal anti-inflammatory drugs. Lancet *343*, 769-772 (1994).
40. Begaud, B., Chaslerie, A., Carne, X., et al., Upper gastrointestinal bleeding associated with analgesics and NSAID use: a case-control study. J. Rheum. *20*, 1443–1444 (1993).
41. Holvoet, J., Terriere, L., Van Hee, W., et al., Relation of upper gastrointestinal bleeding to non-steroidal anti-inflammatory drugs and aspirin: a case-control study. Gut *32*, 730–734 (1991).
42. Lanza, L.L., Walker, A.M., Bortnichak, E.A., Dreyer, N.A., Peptic ulcer and gastrointestinal hemorrhage associated with nonsteroidal anti-inflammatory drug use in patients younger than 65 years. Arch. Intern. Med. *155*, 1371–1377 (1995).
43. Levy, M., Miller, D.R., Kaufman, D.W., et al., Major upper gastrointestinal tract bleeding: relation to the use of aspirin and other nonnarcotic analgesics. Arch. Intern. Med. *148*, 281–285 (1988).
44. Weil, J., Colin-Jones, .D, Langman, M., et al., Prophylactic aspirin and risk of peptic ulcer bleeding. Br. Med. J. *310*, 827–830 (1995).
45. Carson, J.L., Strom, B.L., Soper, K.A., West, S.L., Morse, M.L., The association of nonsteroidal anti-inflammatory drugs with upper gastrointestinal tract bleeding. Arch. Intern. Med. *147*, 85–88 (1987).

46. Graham, D.Y., Smith, J.L., Dobbs, S.M., Gastric adaptation occurs with aspirin adminis-
    tration in man. Dig. Dis. Sci. *28*, 1–6. (1983)
47. Shorrock, C.J., Rees, W.D.W., Mucosal adaptation to indomethacin induced gastric dam-
    age in man – studies on morphology, blood flow, and prostaglandin E2 metabolism. Gut.
    33, 164–169 (1992).
48. Graham, D.Y., Smith, J.L., Spjut, H.J., Torres, E., Gastric adaptation – studies in humans
    during continuous aspirin administration. Gastroenterol. *95*, 327–333 (1988).
49. Shorrock, C.J., Prescott, R.J., Rees, W.D.W., The effects of indomethacin on gastroduo-
    denal morphology and mucosal pH gradient in the healthy human stomach.
    Gastroenterol. *99*, 334–339 (1990).